Essentials
of
FIRST AID

AN AUTHORISED MANUAL OF

St. John Ambulance

SECOND EDITION
1972

SECOND EDITION

First Impression	150,000	1972
Second Impression	100,000	1974
Third Impression	50,000	1976
Fourth Impression	50,000	1977
Fifth Impression	50,000	1978
Sixth Impression	50,000	1980
Seventh Impression	50,000	1980

Printed in England by Henry Burt & Son Ltd., Bedford

Foreword

The Essentials of First Aid provides a course of instruction covering the same ground as the full Standard First Aid Course, and leading to the award of a Certificate not amounting to the statutory Adult qualification. Because of this, the arrangements for lecturing and examining are less stringent than for the senior qualification. It has, therefore, proved exceedingly popular with members of the public seeking a first instruction to the subject and to overseas users. A number of translations have been prepared. It is also used by several industries for first-year entrants. The Certificate is required of all who join the Cadet Branch of the St. John Ambulance Brigade.

With these factors in mind, care has been taken in the present edition to ensure that the user, who intended to pursue a serious First Aid career, is led by an easy and natural transition, to the Authorized First Aid Manual issued jointly by St. John Ambulance, the St. Andrew's Ambulance Association and the British Red Cross Society.

Of the many notable services to St. John Ambulance attributable to my predecessor, Professor H. C. Stewart, the authorship of this publication ranks high.

P. A. LINGARD
Director-General

22nd August, 1978

Contents

Syllabus

The Essentials of First Aid, provides an introductory course of instruction, leading to a Certificate in First Aid, which does not amount to the statutory or standard First Aid Certificate recognized officially in various legislation.

The course, however, embraces much of the standard course contained in the Authorised First Aid Manual of the three Voluntary Aid Societies, and a close study of this book will provide a good grounding for the senior Manual. Traditionally, the course has been designed to cover six weekly sessions of about $2-2\frac{1}{2}$ hours, divided roughly between theoretical and practical instruction. In practice, however, the course may be delivered under any arrangement decided locally, and for day-release purposes may be given over two full days of instruction.

The qualifications for lecturers and examiners are as set out in the Regulations for Classes of St. John Ambulance, which are sent post free on application to the Registrar, St. John Ambulance Association and Brigade, 1 Grosvenor Crescent, SW1, or to any local Association Centre.

SESSION 1

Theory	Principles and Practice of First Aid	chapter 1
	Structure and Functions of the body	chapter 2
Practical	Dressings and Bandages	chapter 3

SESSION 2

Theory	Respiration and asphyxia	
Practical	Emergency resuscitation and the recovery position	chapter 4

SESSION 3

Theory	Circulation of the blood	chapter 5
	Wounds and bleeding and circulatory failure	chapter 6
	Shock	chapter 7
Practical	Control of bleeding. Pressure points	

SESSION 4

Theory   Injuries to bones   chapter 8
                 Injuries to muscles, ligaments and joints   chapter 9
Practical   Management of fractures, dislocations

SESSION 5

Theory   The nervous system and unconsciousness   chapter 10
                 Burns and scalds   chapter 11
                 Poisoning   chapter 12
Practical   Management of fractures and spinal injuries

SESSION 6

Theory   Miscellaneous conditions   chapter 13
                 Handling and transport of injured persons   chapter 14
                 Road accidents   appendix
Practical   Resuscitation, recovery position, dressings
                 and bandages
                 Pressure points

6

CHAPTER ONE

The principles and practice of First Aid

First Aid is the skilled application of accepted principles of treatment on the occurrence of an injury or in the case of sudden illness, using facilities or materials available at the time. It is the approved method of treating a casualty until placed, if necessary, in the care of a doctor or removed to hospital.

First aid treatment is given to a casualty —
— to sustain life;
— to prevent his condition from becoming worse;
— to promote recovery.

First Aider's responsibility

This ends when the casualty is handed over to the care of a doctor, a nurse or other responsible person. The First Aider should not leave until he has made his report to the person who takes charge, and has ascertained whether he could be of any further help.

In some countries where there are areas which are sparsely populated, or in other special circumstances, the First Aider may have to remain many hours, or more exceptionally a few days, with the casualty. Then the redressing of injuries and other after-care treatment procedures may become his responsibility, because there may be no one else available or knowledgeable enough to carry them out.

Instruction in First Aid

This manual teaches standard methods of treatment for definite conditions or adopts recognised principles. The First Aider will find that the same injuries vary considerably in different persons and under different circumstances, and he must always be prepared to adapt himself to any variation from the average.

7

1. TAKE PROMPT ACTION

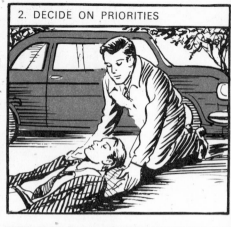

2. DECIDE ON PRIORITIES

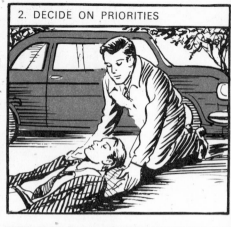

3. REMOVE TO SHELTER

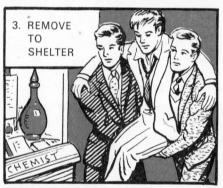

4. IMPROVISE SHELTER

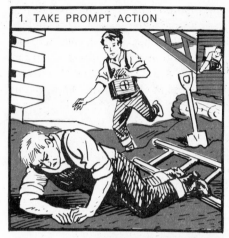

5. ADEQUATE LIGHTING

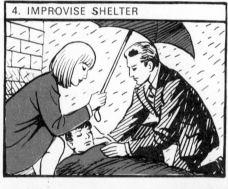

6. KEEP BACK CROWD

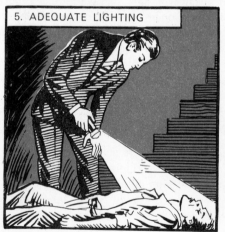

Remember at all times the importance of *Common Sense in First Aid* as an addition to the actual knowledge of the subject. This and other First Aid Manuals of necessity usually consider for treatment only one condition at a time. However, in real life, and consequently in First Aid Competitions also, it will be found that serious accidents rarely produce only a single injury. Frequently, two injuries or more occur so that the correct treatment of one may interfere with the correct treatment of the other. One injury may require the casualty placed on his back but another that he should be placed in the recovery position (see page 12). In such circumstances, the First Aider must decide which injury is the most serious or needs the most urgent treatment and treat that one in the correct way and then deal with the second injury as correctly as possible under the conflicting circumstances.

The scope of First Aid

This consists of four parts:

1. **Assessing** the situation.

2. **Diagnosing** what is wrong with the casualty.

3. Giving immediate and appropriate **treatment**.

4. **Disposing of the casualty** to doctor, hospital or home, according to the seriousness of his condition.

Assessing the situation

Be calm and take charge.
Give confidence to the casualty — talk to him, listen to him and reassure him.
Ensure safety of casualty and yourself.
Guard against any further casualties arising. In the case of —
road accidents — instruct someone to control traffic;
fire and collapsing buildings — move the casualty to safety;
gas and poisonous fumes — turn off or prevent at source;
electrocution — switch off the current: take precautions against electric shock.

Get others to help.
Make use of bystanders — keep them occupied, the more they are given to do, the less they will interfere. They should be used to —
— telephone for the ambulance, police and other services;
— keep back any crowds;
— assist with the control of traffic;
— assist, if necessary, with the actual treatment.

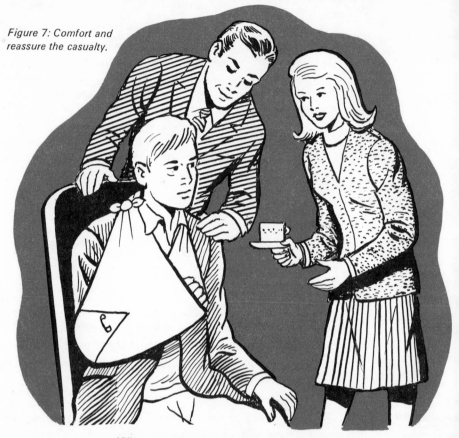

Figure 7: Comfort and reassure the casualty.

When sending bystanders to telephone, make sure that they understand the message to be sent: write it down, if possible, but in any case ask them to repeat the message before actually sending it. See that they report back to you.

Diagnosis

In arriving at a diagnosis the First Aider is guided by —

History of the case — report furnished by the conscious casualty or by persons present as to how the accident happened or illness began;

Symptoms — details of his sensations obtained from the casualty when conscious;

Signs — obtained by a complete examination of the casualty.

Use all your senses to obtain maximum information — look, speak, listen, feel and smell.

10

Conscious casualty

If casualty is conscious –
– ask him if he has pain and where it is: examine that part first;
– handle injured parts gently but firmly;
– make sure there are no other injuries present which may be masked by pain, by asking the casualty if he thinks there is anything else wrong and by checking for tenderness and bleeding.

Examine the casualty carefully in a regular and methodical manner by running your hands gently but firmly over all parts of the body. Start at the head and neck, then check the spine and trunk, the upper limbs, and the lower limbs. Always compare the abnormal side with the normal.

The First Aider need only remove enough of the casualty's clothing to expose the injuries and to treat them.
Then check –
– colour of the skin
– the nature of the breathing – listen to it: smell the breath
– the pulse – count it, note its strength and rhythm
– the temperature of the body – whether it is hot or cold to the touch.

Unconscious casualty

If the casualty is unconscious –
– the task is much more difficult and a thorough detailed examination is necessary, as no symptoms are available to help.
– Note if breathing is present. If absent immediately commence artificial respiration.
– Examine over and under the casualty for dampness which might indicate bleeding or incontinence. Stop any serious bleeding before proceeding further with the examination. Bear in mind the possibility of internal bleeding.

Establish the cause of unconsciousness by examining the –
– *breathing* – rate and depth
– *pulse* – rate and character
– *face and skin* – colour, temperature and condition
– *pupils of the eyes* – size, re-action
– *head* – for injury
– *ears, eyes, nose and mouth* – for blood or other signs
– *whole body* – for signs of injury.

11

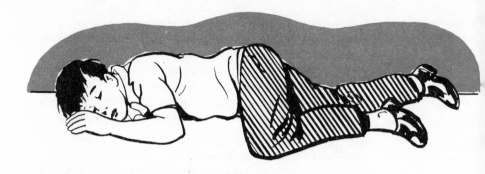

Figure 8: The recovery position (see Page 14).

Multiple casualties

Where there is more than one casualty, the First Aider must decide by rapid assessment, which one should receive priority of treatment.

Immediately placing any unconscious casualty in the recovery position, especially if you are working alone and before attending to any other; effect temporary control of continuous severe bleeding with the assistance of the casualty or by a bystander, if available.

Remember, the noisiest casualty is rarely the most severely injured.

Treatment

The most urgent matters are –

– To apply artificial respiration if the casualty is not breathing. If in doubt as to whether the casualty is alive or not, continue treatment until medical aid is available or a stiffening of the muscles after death (rigor mortis) commences.

– To control bleeding.

– To maintain a clear airway by correctly positioning the casualty.

– To determine the level of consciousness, if he is not fully conscious.

The most important procedures to prevent the condition becoming worse are –

– To place the casualty in the most comfortable position consistent with the requirements of treatment.

– To dress wounds.

– To immobilise fractures and large wounds.

12

The most helpful measures in promoting recovery are –
– To relieve the casualty of anxiety and promote his confidence.
– To relieve him of pain and discomfort.
– To protect him from cold.
– To handle gently so as to do no harm.

Disposal

After treatment has been given, the casualty may be –
– sent to hospital by ambulance;
– handed over to the care of a doctor, nurse or other responsible person;
– taken into a nearby house or shelter to await the arrival of ambulance or doctor; or
– allowed to go home and told to seek medical advice, if necessary.

Do not send anyone home unaccompanied who has been *unconscious*, if only for a short period, or is badly *shocked*.

A message explaining the circumstances and treatment given should accompany the casualty when sent to hospital or to a doctor. If necessary, accompany the casualty and make a personal report.

Notify the nearest relative and any other person or organisation (e.g. his employer) that should be told.

In serious outdoor accidents the police should always be sent for or notified.

Removal of clothing

It is often necessary to remove clothing to expose injuries and to treat them properly. Such removal should be done with a minimum of disturbance to the casualty and clothing, and only as much as is actually necessary. Clothing should not be damaged unnecessarily.

Method

Coat
Raise the casualty and slip the coat over his shoulders; then remove from the sound side first. If necessary slit up the seam of the sleeve on the injured side.

Shirt and vest
Remove as for a coat. If necessary slit the shirt down the front.

13

Trousers

Pull down from the waist or raise trouser leg as required. If necessary slit up the seam.

Boot or shoe

Steady the ankle, undo or cut the laces and remove carefully.

Socks

If difficult to remove, insert two fingers between the sock and the leg, raise the edge of the sock and cut it between your fingers.

Turning a casualty

To turn a casualty when lying on his back into the **Recovery position** (previously known as the coma position) —

1. Kneel beside him and place both his arms close to his body; cross his far leg over his near leg; protect his face with one of your hands; gently turn the casualty on to his side. This may be done by grasping the casualty's clothing at the hip.

2. Draw up the upper arm until it makes a right angle to the body and bend the elbow.

3. Draw up the upper leg until the thigh makes a right angle to the body and bend the knee.

4. Draw out the underneath arm gently backwards to extend it slightly behind his back.

5. Bend the undermost knee slightly (see figure 8).

The effect of placing the limbs in this manner provides the necessary stability to keep the casualty comfortable in the **recovery position.**

If the casualty is a heavy person, two hands may be necessary to grasp the clothing and in this instance the First Aider should kneel at the side of the casualty so that when he is turned his face will rest against the First Aider's knees. If bystanders are present make use of them to protect the casualty's face and assist with the turning.

Procedure at road accidents

Avoid further injury to the casualty, protect bystanders and yourself.

Immediate action

Do not run to the car and start pulling the injured out— unnecessary movement often makes the injuries worse.

Switch off the car engine; apply the hand brake or use wheel chocks, if necessary.

Impose a 'No Smoking' ban.

Send someone to flag down the traffic on both sides of the accident, *at least 300 yards* (or metres) away.

Stop passing cars and ask drivers to telephone for the police (using the 999 system where applicable), give the exact location of the accident, number of injured, the number and types of vehicles involved. It is wise to send one car in each direction with this information. The police will inform other services as required.

Dealing with the victims

Inside the vehicle

Wherever possible, leave the removal of the severely injured casualties to the specially trained personnel of the Emergency Services.

If it is essential to remove the casualty, owing to the risk of fire, etc., ensure that there is adequate help to support all parts of the casualty and aim to make the removal in one smooth continuous operation.

The priorities of treatment in road accidents should be directed at —

(i) breathing
(ii) bleeding
(iii) unconsciousness.

Ensure an open airway at all times.

Outside the vehicle

If it is necessary to move the injured person urgently from the roadway, it should be done as carefully and as gently as possible.

Note the exact position of the casualty, also the time and place of the accident, as this information will be required by the police.

If a person is trapped under a car and has to be moved owing to the possibility of fire, etc., before the arrival of the Emergency Services, make sure that the vehicle is carefully immobilised. If one side of the car is lifted ensure you are not pushing the other side down onto someone else.

15

General   If there are several casualties, the First Aider must decide by rapid assessment which one should receive priority of treatment. See 'Multiple casualties' on page 12.

Summary of priorities in first aid

Act quickly, quietly and methodically, giving priority to the most urgent conditions.

Ensure that there is no further danger to the casualty or yourself.

If breathing has stopped, or is failing, clear the airway and, if necessary, start artificial respiration.

Control bleeding.

Determine the level of consciousness.

Consider the possibility of poisoning.

Give re-assurance as necessary to the casualty and to those around and so help to lessen anxiety.

Guard against shock (see page 75).

Position the casualty correctly.

Before moving the casualty, immobilise fractures and large wounds.

Arrange without delay for the careful conveyance of the casualty, if necessary, to the care of his doctor or to a hospital.

Watch and record any changes in the condition of the casualty.

Do not attempt too much.

Do not allow people to crowd round: this hinders first aid and may cause the casualty anxiety or embarrassment.

Do not remove clothing unnecessarily.

Do not give anything by the mouth to a casualty who is unconscious, who has a suspected internal injury, or who may shortly need an anaesthetic.

First Aider – definition and duty

Definition   The term First Aider was first used in 1894 by the Voluntary First Aid Organisations to denote a person who has been trained by and received a Certificate from an authorised association that 'he or she is qualified to render First Aid'.

The St. John Ambulance Association issues such a certificate to candidates successful in an examination conducted by specially appointed Medical Practitioners at the end of a course of theoretical and practical work.

The Certificate has a limited validity of three years.

The general public today demand that such volunteers be —
— Highly trained.
— Regularly examined.
— Kept up-to-date in knowledge and skill.

As you will often have their lives in your hands, they have a right to expect the highest standards of efficiency.

Duty

In order to render the skilled assistance required the First Aider must deploy all his resources with intelligence.

He must be —

Observant — that he may note the causes and signs of injury and search for special information (treatment cards, etc.) which may have a bearing on the diagnosis.

Tactful — that he may, without thoughtless questions, learn the symptoms and history of the case, and secure the confidence of the casualty and the bystanders in the treatment of the casualty.

Resourceful — that he may use to the best advantage whoever and whatever is at hand to prevent further damage and to assist Nature's efforts to repair the situation, improvising where ideal conditions may not exist.

Dextrous — that he may handle a casualty without causing unnecessary pain, and use appliances efficiently, quickly and neatly.

Explicit — that he may give clear instructions to the casualty and/or the bystanders how best to assist him.

Discriminating — that he may decide which of several casualties and injuries should be treated first, and where modification of the correct treatment, as the result of common sense, may be necessary.

Persevering — that he may continue his efforts, though not at first successful, until relieved by a superior medical authority, or death of the casualty is undoubted.

Sympathetic – that he may give real comfort and encouragement to the suffering, always remembering the first principles of humanity.

These qualifications were in times past shown as the Beatitudes surrounding the Eight-pointed Cross, and in tribute and commemoration of our predecessors we reproduce it on this page.

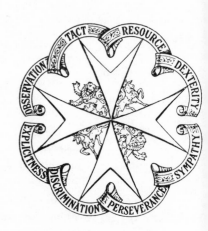

Figure 9:
The eight pointed
ambulance cross.

CHAPTER TWO

Structure and functions of the body

In order to understand the principles of First Aid, it is necessary to know something of the structure of the body and the functions of the more important organs and systems.

The skeleton

The body is built on a bone framework called the **skeleton,** which –
– gives it shape and firmness;
– provides levers for the muscles to work;
– gives protection to important organs in the skull, chest and abdomen.

The skull

The rounded part of the skull forms a rigid protection for the brain. Through the base of the skull pass blood vessels and nerves, including the mass of nerve fibres called the spinal cord, which passes down the spinal canal contained in the vertebral column.

The bones of the face, with the exception of the lower jaw, are firmly united and form, together with the bones of the skull, cavities for the nose and eye sockets. The upper jaw bone has sockets for the upper teeth. The lower jaw bone, the only movable part of the skull, consists of a horizontal portion in which are the sockets for the lower teeth, two vertical portions terminating and hinging on to each side of the base of the skull in front of the ear. The junction of the horizontal and vertical portions is known as 'the angle of the jaw'.

Spine or back-bone (vertebral column)

The spine is formed by thirty-three bones called *vertebrae.* Each is known as a *vertebra.*

The vertebrae are grouped in regions in each of which they

19

The Skeleton and Main Arteries

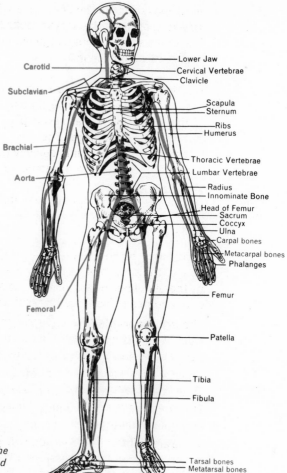

Carotid
Subclavian
Brachial
Aorta
Femoral

Lower Jaw
Cervical Vertebrae
Clavicle
Scapula
Sternum
Ribs
Humerus
Thoracic Vertebrae
Lumbar Vertebrae
Radius
Innominate Bone
Head of Femur
Sacrum
Coccyx
Ulna
Carpal bones
Metacarpal bones
Phalanges
Femur
Patella
Tibia
Fibula
Tarsal bones
Metatarsal bones
Phalanges

Figure 10: The skeleton.

In describing the body it is presumed to be erect with the arms hanging by the side and the palm of the left hand directed forward.

are known by numbers counting downwards —
– in the neck: seven *cervical* vertebrae;
– in the back: twelve *thoracic* vertebrae, to which are attached the ribs;
– in the loin: five *lumbar* vertebrae;
– the rump-bone (*sacrum*): five sacral vertebrae, fused together in adults;
– the tail-bone (*coccyx*): four vertebrae fused together.

Between the bodies of the vertebrae in the first three regions there are thick pieces of cartilage, known as discs, which allow movement of the spine as a whole and help to absorb the shock of any sudden force applied to the vertebral column. The whole spine is bound together by bands of strong fibrous tissues called ligaments.

Ribs and breastbone (sternum)

The ribs consist of twelve pairs of curved bones extending from the thoracic vertebrae on each side round to the front of the body, the upper seven pairs being attached to the breastbone by cartilage. The next three pairs are attached by cartilage to the rib immediately above them: the last two pairs are unattached in front and are know as 'floating ribs'.

Shoulder and upper limbs

The bones of the shoulder are the collar-bone (*clavicle*), the shoulder-blade (*scapula*) and the upper arm bone (*humerus*).

The **collar-bone** (*clavicle*) can be felt between the upper part of the breastbone and the outer part of the upper part of the shoulder. It is a narrow curved bone which forms a strut and maintains the upper limb away from the chest.

The **shoulder-blade** (*scapula*) lies at the upper and outer side of the back of the chest, and forms joints with the collar-bone and the bone of the upper arm.

The bones of the upper limb are –
One in the **upper arm** (*humerus*) and two bones in the **forearm** (*radius* and *ulna*) which allow for the turning action of the wrist.

There are eight small *carpal* bones at the **wrist**; five *metacarpal* bones forming the framework of the palm of the **hand**, which supports the bones of the fingers and thumbs. There are three small bones (*phalanges*) in each **finger** and two in each **thumb.**

Pelvis and lower limbs

The **pelvis** is the large basin-like mass of bone, attached to the lower part of the spine, and which contains the lower abdominal contents and provides sockets for the hip joints.

The **thigh-bone** (*femur*), reaching from the hip to the knee, is the longest and strongest bone in the body. It broadens out at its lower end to form part of the **knee-joint.**

The **knee-cap** (*patella*) is a small triangular bone lying in front of and protecting the knee-joint.

Bones of the leg, two in number, extend from the knee to the ankle, the long thin bone (*fibula*) lying on the outer side of the thicker **shin-bone** (*tibia*).

The bones of the **foot** consist of seven *tarsal* bones in the ankle, five *metatarsal* bones in the instep, supporting the bones of the toes, which have three small bones (*phalanges*) in each, except the big toe which has two.

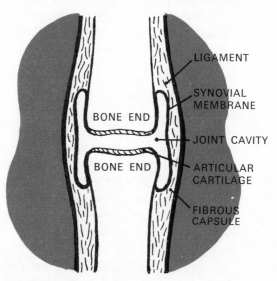

LIGAMENT

SYNOVIAL MEMBRANE

BONE END

JOINT CAVITY

BONE END

ARTICULAR CARTILAGE

FIBROUS CAPSULE

Figure 11: Joint.

Joints

Joints are formed by the junction of two or more bones. These may be immovable allowing no movement such as joints between the bones forming the dome of the skull, or they may be movable. In this case the ends of the bones are covered with *cartilage*, held together by strong bands of tissue called *ligaments* and enclosed in a bag known as a *capsule*, inside of which is a lining which secretes fluid to act as a lubricant. The movable joints are of three types –

– The *ball and socket*, formed by the rounded head of one bone fitting into the cup-shaped cavity of another bone, and allowing free movement, such as found in the shoulder and hip joints.

– *Hinged joints,* in which the surface of the bones are moulded to each other so that they can only move in one plane: bending or straightening. The elbow is a typical example of this.

– *Slightly movable joints,* which are limited in the extent of their movement, e.g. the foot.

Inside the knee-joint there are two pieces of cartilage. In sudden wrenches, such as may happen in football or other games, these cartilages may be torn and produce considerable pain.

The tissues

The body is built up of different kinds of materials called 'tissue', which are composed of a multitude of tiny units called 'cells'.

The skin

This covers the whole of the body and protects the underlying structures from injury and infection. Within it are numerous glands which secrete sweat and impurities from the blood and these escape through tiny openings on the surface of the skin, thus helping to regulate the temperature of the body.

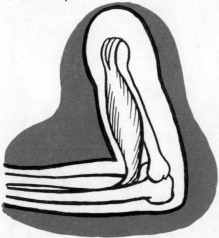

Figure 12: Muscles.

Muscles

These move various parts of the body. One type is known as the **'voluntary muscles'** and are attached to bones. When they are stimulated to contract, they produce either

23

flexion (bending) or extension (straightening) of the parts to which they are attached. Being under the control of the will they will help in movement when we wish.

Involuntary muscles are found in the heart and blood vessels, the walls of the stomach, intestines, and most of the internal organs. These produce movements which are not under the control of our will, but continue their work at all times.

The trunk and its contents

The trunk is divided by a large arched muscular partition (*diaphragm*) into two cavities – the upper, the chest (*thorax*) and the lower (*abdomen*).

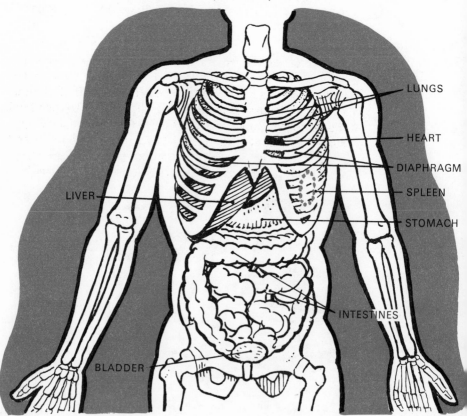

Figure 13: The trunk and its contents.

Chest cavity

The chest cavity, bounded in front by the breastbone, behind by the thoracic vertebrae, below by the diaphragm, and encircled by the ribs, contains the heart, major blood vessels, the lungs, and the gullet.

Abdominal cavity

The lower cavity, bounded above by the diaphragm, below by the pelvis, behind by the lumbar vertebrae and in front and at the sides by muscular walls, contains several important organs — the *liver*, on the right side; the *spleen* under the ribs on the upper part of the left side; the *stomach*, just below the diaphragm on the left side; the *pancreas* behind the stomach. The *intestines* fill the greater part of the cavity of the abdomen. Two *kidneys* are at the back in the region of the loins, whilst the *bladder* lies to the front of the pelvis.

Functions of the body

The body works very much like an internal combustion engine. We feed it with food and fluid which are digested and carried to the tissues of the body by means of the bloodstream. In the tissues the digested matter meets oxygen from the air we breathe into the lungs, the resulting changes supply the body with materials for maintaining life and producing all its activities. The waste is got rid of through the lungs, skin, bladder and bowels.

CHAPTER THREE

Dressings and bandages

Dressings

A dressing is a protective covering applied to a wound to –
– prevent infection;
– absorb discharge;
– control bleeding;
– avoid further injury.

An efficient dressing should be *sterile* (germ free) and have a high degree of porosity to allow for oozing and sweating.

Adhesive dressings

These sterile dressings are of different kinds and consist of a pad of absorbent gauze or cellulose, held in place by a layer of adhesive material. The surrounding skin must be dry before application and all the edges of the dressing pressed firmly down.

Sterile adhesive dressings are supplied in paper or plastic covers.

Non-adhesive dressings

Prepared (standard) sterile dressing. The dressing consists of layers of gauze covered by a pad of cotton wool with an attached roller bandage to hold it in position. The dressing is enclosed and sealed in protective covering and is supplied in various sizes.

Gauze dressing. Gauze in layers is commonly used as a dressing for large wounds, as it is very absorbent, soft and pliable. It is liable to adhere to the wound: however, this may assist the clotting of blood. The dressing should be covered by one or more layers of cotton wool.

Improvised dressing. These can be made from any clean, soft, absorbent material such as the inside of a clean handkerchief, a piece of linen, a clean paper handkerchief or cellulose tissue. They should be covered and retained in position by such materials as are available.

Application of dressings

Great care must be taken in handling and applying dressings. If possible, wash your hands thoroughly.

Avoid touching any part of the wound with the fingers or any part of the dressing which will be in contact with the wound.

Do not talk or cough over the wound or the dressing.

Dressings must be covered with adequate pads of cotton wool, extending well beyond them and retained in position by a bandage or strapping.

If a dressing adheres to the wound, careful soaking is required before removal.

Bandages

These are made from flannel, calico, elastic net or special paper. They can be improvised by any of the above materials, or from stockings, ties, scarves, belts, etc.

Bandages are used to —
— maintain direct pressure over a dressing to control bleeding;
— retain dressings and splints in position;
— prevent or reduce swelling;
— provide support for a limb or joint;
— restrict movement;
— assist in lifting and carrying casualties.

Bandages should **not** be used for padding when other materials are available.

Bandages should be applied firmly enough to keep dressing and splints in position, but not so tightly as to cause injury to the part or to impede the circulation of the blood. A bluish tinge of the finger or toe nails may be a danger sign that the bandages are too tight: loss of sensation is another sign.

The triangular bandage

The triangular bandage is made by cutting a piece of material (linen, calico or even strong paper) not less than one yard (one metre) square, diagonally into two, thus producing two bandages.

Uses

As a whole cloth in the form of a sling or opened to its full extent for keeping a dressing in position (Fig. 14).

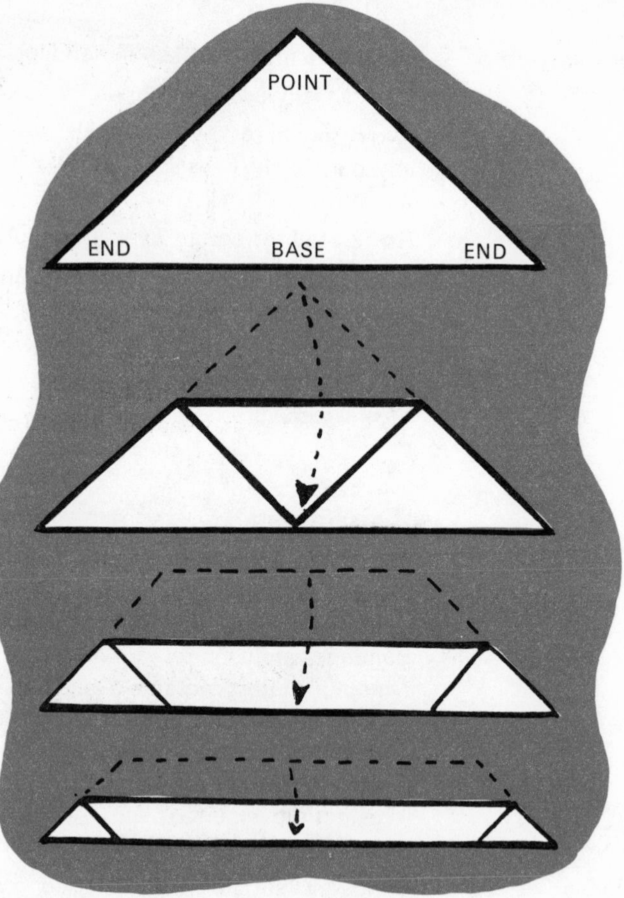

Figure 14:
The triangular bandage.

Figure 15:
Folded once (seldom used).

Figure 16:
Folded twice – used
as a broad bandage.

Figure 17:
Folded three times –
used as a narrow bandage.

POINT

END   BASE   END

As a broad bandage, made by bringing the point down to the centre of the base and then folding the bandage again in the same direction (Figs. 15 and 16).

As a narrow bandage, made by folding the broad bandage once again in the same direction (Fig. 17).

As a ring pad, made by passing one end of a narrow bandage once or twice round the fingers, then bringing the other end of the bandage through the loop and continue to pass it through and through until the whole bandage is used and a firm ring is made (Fig. 18).

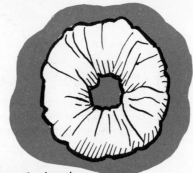

Figure 18:
The triangular bandage
as a ring pad.

To tie a triangular bandage
The bandage should be tied with a reef-knot, which does not slip, is flat and easy to untie. To tie a reef-knot, put left over right and right over left (Fig. 19).

Figure 19:
The reef knot.

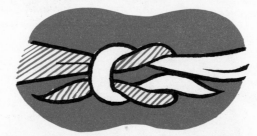

If the bandage or knot is likely to cause discomfort, a pad must be placed between the bandage or knot and the body.

After the knot is tied, the ends of the bandage should be tucked neatly out of sight.

When not in use the triangular bandage should be folded narrow and the ends turned over towards the middle (Fig. 20).

Figure 20:
The triangular bandage
folded for storage.

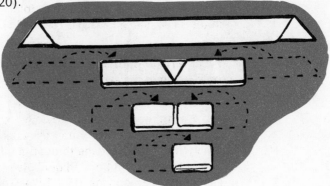

Slings

Slings are used when necessary to afford support and protection to the upper limb.

Arm sling

To support the forearm and hand where there are wounds and injuries to the upper limb and in some cases of fractured ribs. It is only affective when the casualty is sitting or standing.

Method. Support the forearm on the injured side, wrist and hand a little higher than the elbow. Place an open triangular bandage **between** the chest and the forearm, with the point stretching beyond the elbow. Carry the upper end **over** the shoulder on the uninjured side and round the neck to the front of the injured side. Bring the lower end of the bandage up over the hand and forearm and tie off in

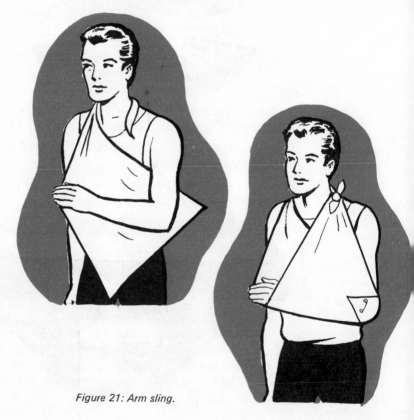

Figure 21: Arm sling.

front of the hollow above the collar-bone. Bring the point forward and secure in the front of the bandage with a safety pin (Fig. 21). The base of the bandage should be at the root of the little finger, so that all the fingers are exposed for observation. If circulation is impeded –

(a) the position of the hand should be altered,

(b) an adjustment made of the bandage, *or*

(c) the sling removed.

Triangular (St. John) sling

To support the hand and forearm in a well-raised position, as in the case of a hand injury or severely fractured ribs.

Method. The forearm on the injured side is supported across the chest with the fingers pointing to the shoulder on the opposite side. Place an open triangular bandage **over** the forearm and hand with the point extending well beyond the elbow and its upper end over the shoulder on the sound side. Gently ease the base of the bandage under the forearm, hand and elbow and carry the lower end round the back and on to

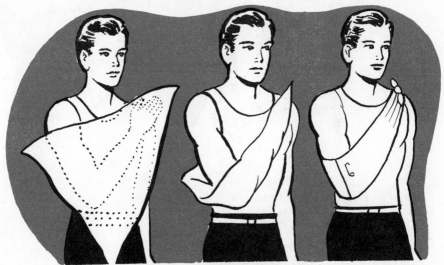

Figure 22: Triangular (St. John) sling.

the front of the sound shoulder. Gently adjust the height of the sling and tie the ends off in the hollow above the collar-bone on the uninjured side. Tuck the point of the bandage between the forearm and the bandage and secure with a safety pin. (Fig. 22).

Application of the triangular bandage

In the following applications, a narrow hem should be turned up along the inside of the base of the bandage.

Scalp and head   Stand behind the casualty and place the centre of the hem of the bandage over the forehead with the point hanging down at the back of the head. Carry the ends round the head just above the ears, cross them over the point of the bandage near the nape of the neck, and bring them forward round the head over the ears. Tie off on the forehead, close to the hem of the bandage. Draw the point down and fold it up and secure with a safety pin (Fig. 23).

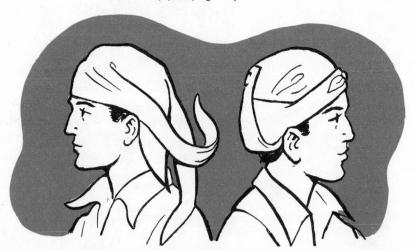

Figure 23: Scalp bandage.

Chest (front)   Stand in front of the casualty and place the centre of the bandage over the dressing with the point over the shoulder on the same side. Carry the ends round the body and tie them at the back leaving one long end, which is taken up and tied to the point on the shoulder (Fig. 24).

Chest (back)   Stand behind the casualty and apply the bandage similarly to that as for the front of the chest.

Shoulder   Stand facing the casualty. Place the centre of the bandage over the shoulder with the point towards the ear. Carry the

32

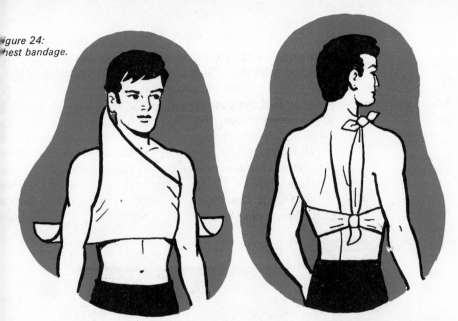

hem of the bandage round the middle of the upper arm, cross the ends and tie them on the outer side. Apply an arm sling. Tuck the point of the bandage under the sling and bring it down over the knot and secure with a safety pin (Fig. 25).

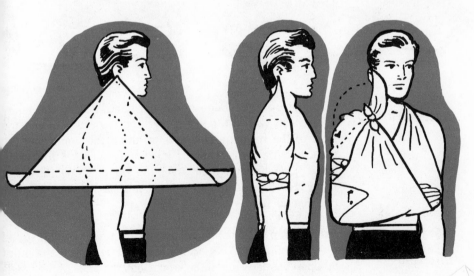

Figure 25: Bandaging the shoulder.

Elbow

Bend the casualty's elbow to a right angle. Lay the point of the bandage on the back of the upper arm and the middle of the base on the back of the forearm. Cross the ends in front of the elbow and then round the upper arm and tie above the elbow. Bring the point down over the knot and secure with a safety pin (Fig. 26).

Figure 26:
Bandaging the elbow.

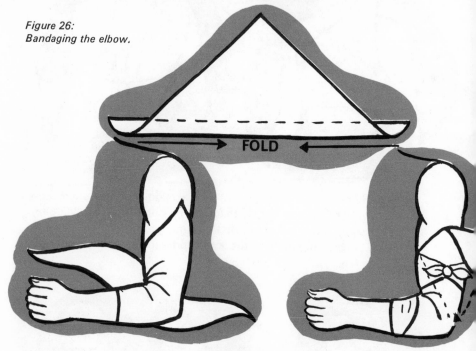

Hand

Place an open bandage under the hand, having the injury uppermost, with the point away from the casualty and the base of the bandage at the wrist. Bring the point over the hand and pass the ends of the bandage round the wrist, cross them and tie them over the point. Draw the point firmly downwards over the knot and secure with a safety pin (Fig. 27).

Hip or groin

Face the hip to be bandaged and tie a narrow bandage round the body with the knot on the injured side. Slip the point of an open bandage under the knot. Carry the ends of the bandage round the thigh, cross them and tie off on the outer side

34

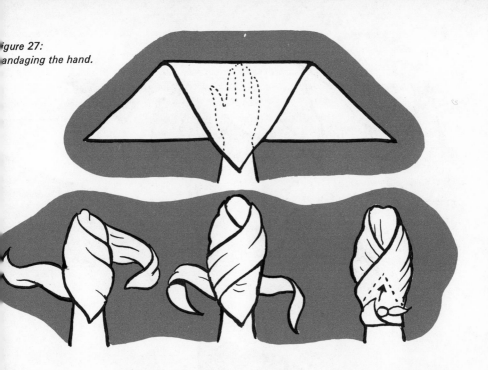

of the thigh. Bring the point over the knot of the narrow bandage and secure with a safety pin (Figs. 28, 29 and 30).

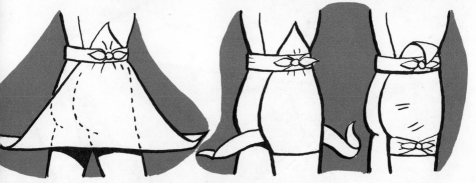

Figures 28, 29 and 30: Bandaging the hip.

Knee

Bend the casualty's knee and lay the point of the bandage on the thigh and the middle of the base just below the knee. Cross the ends of the bandage at the back of the knee, then round the thigh and tie above the knee on the front of the

35

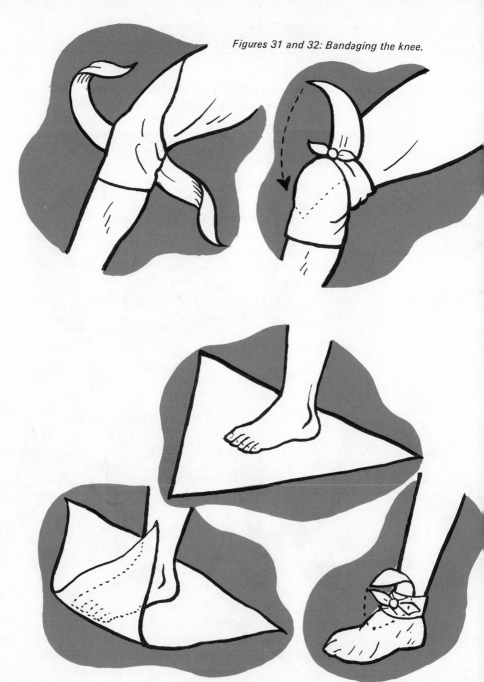

Figures 31 and 32: Bandaging the knee.

Figures 33, 34 and 35: Bandaging the foot.

thigh. Bring the point of the bandage over the knot and secure with a safety pin (Figs. 31 and 32).

Foot

Place the casualty's foot on the centre of an open bandage with the point away from the casualty. Bring the point over the front of the foot. Bring the ends forward so that the heel is covered, cross them, pass the ends round the ankle, cross at the back and tie in front over the point. Draw the point firmly downwards over the knot and secure with a safety pin (Figs. 33, 34 and 35).

Stump

Place the base of a bandage well up on the inside of the stump, the point hanging downwards. Draw up the point over the stump and cross the ends in front over the point. Carry the ends behind the stump, cross them and bring them forward, tying off in front. Draw the point firmly downwards over the knot and secure with a safety pin (Figs. 36, 37 and 38).

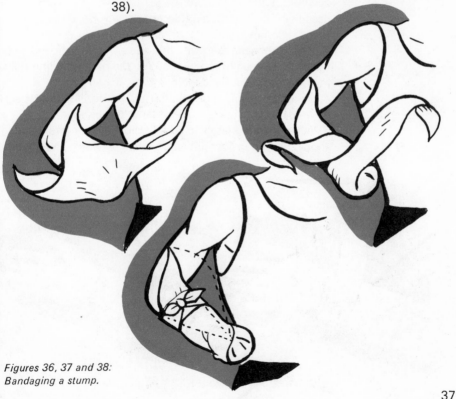

Figures 36, 37 and 38: Bandaging a stump.

Roller bandages

The width of these bandages vary according to the part of the body to be bandaged and the size of the casualty.

Widths normally used are —
– 1 inch (2·5 cm) for the **fingers**
– 2 inch (5 cm) for the **hand**
– 2 to 2½ inches (5 to 6 cm) for the **arm**
– 3 to 3½ inches (7·5 to 9 cm) for the **leg**
– 4 to 6 inches (10 to 15 cm) for the **trunk**.

They are mostly used to keep dressings in position. When partly unrolled the rolled part is called 'the head', and the unrolled part 'the free end'. The bandage should be firmly applied with both edges lying close to the limb.

Application of roller bandages

Rules for the Application of Roller Bandages
1. Use a tightly rolled bandage of suitable width.
2. Support the part to be bandaged. Stand in front of the casualty when bandaging an arm or leg. Bandage a limb in the position in which it is to remain.
3. Hold the bandage with the head uppermost and apply the outer surface of the bandage to the part, unrolling only a few inches of the bandage at a time.
4. Bandage a limb from within outwards and from below upwards; maintaining even pressure throughout.
5. When bandaging a left limb the head of the bandage should be held in the right hand: when bandaging a right limb, in the left.

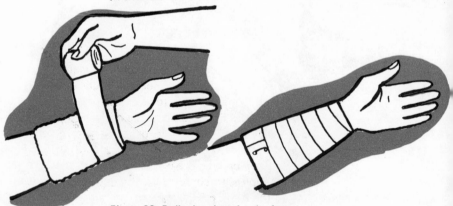

Figure 39: Roller bandage for the forearm.

6. Begin the bandage with a firm oblique turn to fix it and allow each successive turn to cover two-thirds of the previous one, with the free edges lying parallel.

7. Finish off with a straight turn above the part, fold in the end and fasten with a safety pin, adhesive tape or bandage clip.

8. Ensure that the bandage is neither too tight nor too loose.

9. Do not cover the tips of the fingers or toes.

10. Ensure that the circulation of the blood is not impeded. (Figs. 39 and 40).

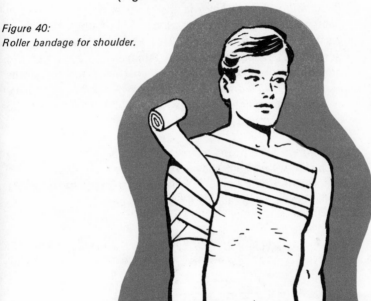

Figure 40:
Roller bandage for shoulder.

Tubular gauze bandage

This is a method of bandaging which is in many ways better and quicker than traditional methods, but it is much more expensive. It consists of a roll of seamless tubular gauze in various sizes to fit numerous parts of the body. It is applied with specially designed applicators of different sizes.

Elasticised net bandage

Elasticised net bandage, a two-way stretch mesh material, is easy to apply and comfortable to wear. It can be used on the head, the trunk or the limbs to retain dressings neatly in position.

39

CHAPTER FOUR

Respiration, asphyxia and emergency resuscitation

Respiration

Respiration or breathing, is the process by which oxygen passes from the air into the blood while carbon dioxide, a waste product, is expelled. This respiratory exchange of gases takes place in the lungs. Atmospheric air which we breathe consists of one fifth oxygen (20%) and four-fifths nitrogen (80%). *There is still 16% oxygen left in the air we breathe out,* which accounts for the effectiveness of the expired-air method of resuscitation.

The lungs

Two lungs fill the greater part of the chest cavity, one on each side of the heart. They are covered by a membrane which is continued as a lining for the inner surfaces of the chest walls. These membranes are called the *pleura.*

Figure 41:
The air entry.

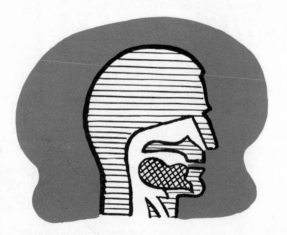

Airway

Air drawn into the lungs enters through the nose and mouth (Fig. 41) and passes down the throat (*pharynx*), through the voice box (*larynx*) to enter the windpipe (*trachea*).

The top of the larynx is protected by a flap *(epiglottis)* which opens for breathing but shuts when food or fluid is being swallowed. In an unconscious casualty this protective mechanism does not function.

In the chest, the trachea divides into two branches, the right and left *bronchus*. Each bronchus passes into a lung where it divides into a great number of small tubes *(bronchioles)* which, after repeated division into smaller and smaller tubes, open finally into numerous minute air-sacs *(alveoli)*. A fine network of blood vessels *(capillaries)* surround the alveoli through which the exchange of gases takes place. (Fig. 42).

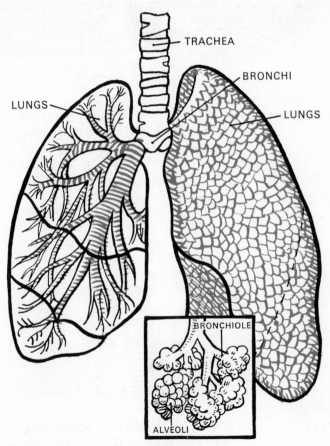

Figure 42: The lungs and bronchioles.

Obstruction of the airway

In an unconscious casualty, the tongue may fall back and block the airway. There is danger of secretion or regurgitated stomach contents entering the windpipe because the epiglottis fails to function.

It is essential to place such casualties in the recovery position.

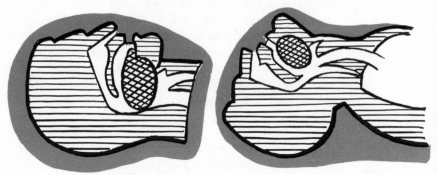

Figure 43: Unconscious person lying on his back – air passages.
Left: The tongue may fall to the back of the throat blocking the airway.
Right: If the neck is extended, the head pressed backwards and the jaw pushed upwards, the tongue moves forward opening the air passages.

Mechanism of respiration

This is controlled by the action of the diaphragm (muscle) and the muscles between the ribs. Air is drawn into the lungs (**inspiration**) and expelled from the lungs (**expiration**). There is a short **pause** between expiration and inspiration. Inspiration is produced by the contraction of the diaphragm, its dome-like centre becomes flattened and draws air in through the air passages. The ribs are raised by the action of the muscles between them and this also increases the size of the chest and helps to suck air inwards.

In expiration, air is forced out through the airway by the diaphragm and the ribs returning to their normal position.

These movements are controlled by the respiratory centres of the brain.

Rate of breathing

This may vary considerably. The average adult at rest breathes 15–18 times per minute. In infants and young children the rate is 24–40 times per minute.

The rate increases if more oxygen is required as in exercise, fever, etc.

Asphyxia

Asphyxia is a condition in which there is lack of oxygen in the blood, and the tissues do not receive an adequate supply because –
– there may be an insufficient amount of oxygen in the air breathed in, *or*
– the lungs and heart have ceased to function effectively.

Asphyxia is one of the most common causes of unconsciousness.

Those affecting the airway and lungs

Fluid, as in some instances of drowning, or from *gas or smoke* in the air passages;
– *compression of the windpipe* by hanging or strangulation;
– *suffocation* (smothering) by pillows, plastic bags, etc.;
– by *obstruction* such as the tongue falling to the back of the throat in an unconscious casualty lying on his back, a mass of food, a foreign body (teeth, blood, vomit), swelling of the tissues within the throat as a result of scalds, stings or infection; *or*
– by *compression of the chest* caused by a fall of earth or sand, crushing against a wall or barrier, pressure in a crowd.

Those affecting the nerves which control respiration

– *Electrical* injury;
– *poisoning* such as barbiturates, morphia and overdose of some common remedies;
– *muscle contraction* as in tetanus;
– *paralysis* as in apoplexy, some nerve illness such as poliomyelitis, or an injury to the spinal cord.

Those affecting the amount of oxygen in the blood

– *Air containing insufficient oxygen* as in smoke-laden buildings, disused shafts, tunnels;
– *change of atmospheric pressure* as in high altitudes and deep sea diving;
– *continuous fits* preventing adequate breathing.

Those preventing the use of oxygen in the body

– *Carbon monoxide poisoning* – household gas (except

43

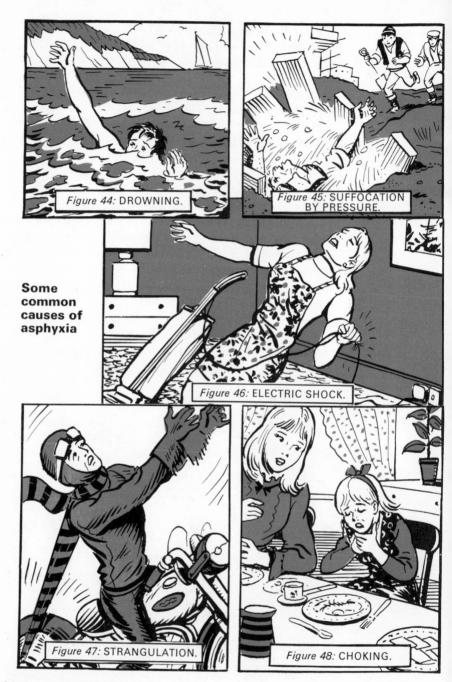

Some common causes of asphyxia

Figure 44: DROWNING.

Figure 45: SUFFOCATION BY PRESSURE.

Figure 46: ELECTRIC SHOCK.

Figure 47: STRANGULATION.

Figure 48: CHOKING.

natural gas from the North Sea), motor exhaust fumes;
– *cyanide poisoning* (prussic acid gas) when the tissues cannot use the oxygen present in the blood.

Signs and symptoms

1. **Breathing** – rate, depth and difficulty increase at first; later becomes noisy with frothing at the mouth, finally stopping.
2. **Congestion** of the head and neck, face and lips.
3. **Consciousness** is gradually lost: fits may occur.

General rules for treatment

The vital needs are –
– **Airway**: open to allow air to reach the lungs;
– **Breathing**: adequate to allow sufficient oxygen to enter the lungs and pass into the blood;
– **Circulation**: sufficient to carry the oxygen-containing blood to the tissues of the body.

Depending on the causes and prevailing circumstances –
1. Remove the casualty from the cause, or the cause from the casualty.
2. Ensure an open airway and adequate air (see page 42).
3. Start emergency resuscitation at once (see below).
4. Use any help available.

Emergency resuscitation

If the brain is deprived of oxygen for more than about four minutes, permanent damage may have been done.

Emergency resuscitation is therefore concerned with –
– the immediate and continued·oxygenation of the blood by inflating the lungs;
– the restarting of the heart to maintain sufficient circulation to ensure that this oxygenated blood reaches the brain and other vital organs (e.g. heart, kidneys).

The most important single factor in any form of respiratory resuscitation is the speed with which the first few inflations can be given.

The urgency is so great that only obvious obstructions should be removed –
– *over the head and face* – plastic bag, pillows;
– *round the neck* – any constriction;
– *in the mouth* – debris, vomit, blood, false teeth or tongue.

Respiratory resuscitation (artificial respiration)

There are several methods of artificial respiration.

The most effective is mouth-to-mouth (mouth-to-nose) and this method can be used by almost all age groups and in almost all circumstances *except –*

– when there is severe injury to the face and mouth;
– when the casualty is pinned in the face-down position;
– if vomiting interferes with respiratory resuscitation.

Waste no time. Start emergency resuscitation immediately. Seconds count.

Figure 49:
Ensure open airway.

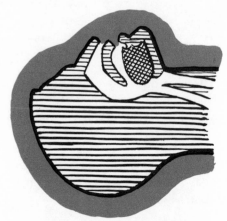

Treatment

If the casualty is not breathing –
1. Ensure he has a good airway –
– support the nape of the neck and press the top of the head so that it is tilted backwards (Fig. 49);
– press the chin upwards (Fig. 50).

These moves extend the head and neck and lift the tongue forward clear of the airway. This is particularly necessary in an unconscious casualty lying on his back when the tongue falls to the back of the throat and blocks the airway.

If the casualty is capable of breathing, this may be all that is necessary: he will gasp and start to breathe. At this point place him in the recovery position.

2. Loosen clothing at neck and waist.

If the casualty does not start to breathe after ensuring a good airway, keep the head tilted backwards and begin mouth-to-mouth (mouth-to-nose) breathing. This is easier to do when the casualty is lying on his back.

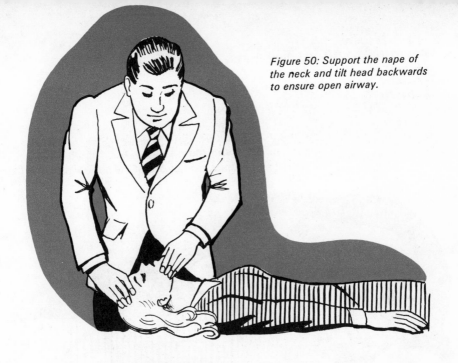

Figure 50: Support the nape of the neck and tilt head backwards to ensure open airway.

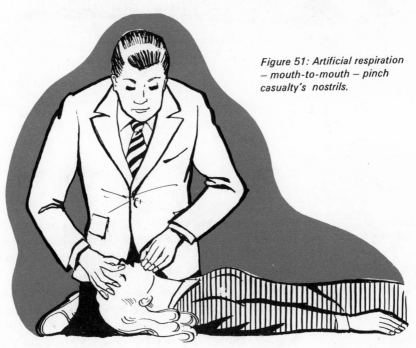

Figure 51: Artificial respiration – mouth-to-mouth – pinch casualty's nostrils.

Mouth-to-mouth method of artificial respiration

In an adult –

– open your mouth wide and take a deep breath;
– pinch the casualty's nostrils together with your fingers (Fig. 51);
– seal your lips round his mouth;
– blow into his lungs until the chest rises (Fig. 52).
– then remove your mouth and watch the chest fall;
– repeat and continue inflations at the natural rate of breathing

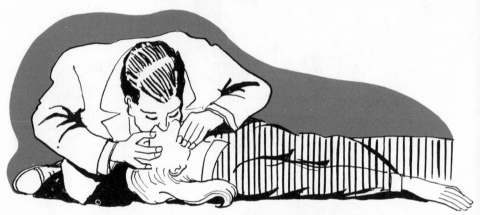

Figure 52: Seal lips round mouth and blow into lungs.

In an infant or young child –

Modify the foregoing instructions by *gently* blowing into his mouth and if necessary seal your lips round his mouth and nose.

Give the first four inflations as rapidly as possible to saturate the blood with oxygen.

General instructions

If the casualty's chest fails to rise, there may be an obstruction. Ensure that his head is tilted well backwards; turn him on his side and thump his back. Check for and remove any foreign matter from the back of the throat (Fig. 53).

If the First Aider cannot make a seal round the casualty's mouth, he should use the mouth-to-nose method. In this case, during inflations, the casualty's mouth should be closed with the thumb of the hand holding the lower jaw (Fig. 54).

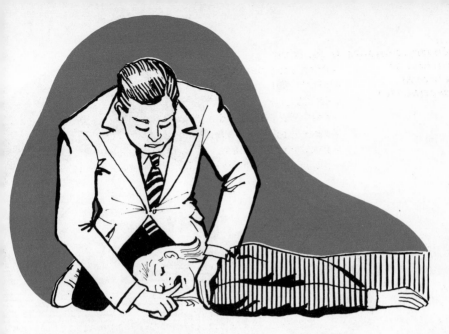

Figure 53: Remove foreign matter from back of throat.

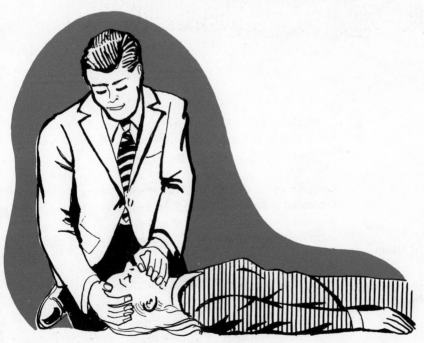

Figure 54: Mouth-to-nose method – close mouth with thumb.

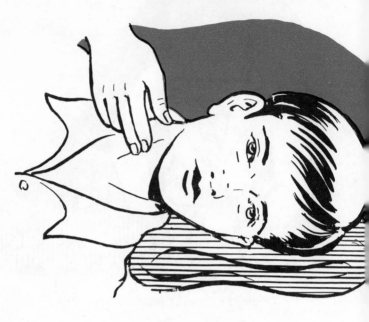

Figure 55:
Feeling the carotid pulse.
Note dilated pupils.

If the heart is NOT beating – the casualty's colour remain
or becomes blue/grey, the pupils are widely dilated, an
the carotid pulse (Fig. 55), cannot be felt –
1. Put the casualty on his back on a firm surface – the floo
2. Strike his chest smartly to the left of the lower part of th
breast-bone with the edge of the hand. This may restart th
heart beating.

If the heart does not beat, start **External Heart Com**
pression *while continuing to give artificial respiration.*

External heart
compression

Method –
1. Take up a position at the side of the casualty.
2. Find the lower half of the breast-bone.
3. Place the heel of your hand on this part of the bone
keeping the palm and fingers off the chest.

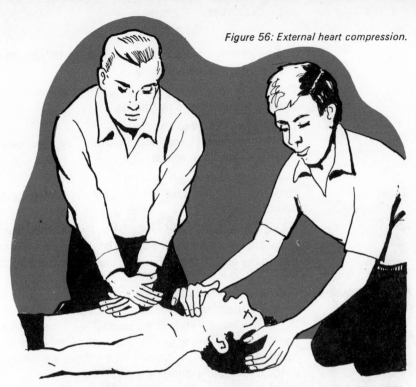

Figure 56: External heart compression.

4. Cover this hand with the heel of the other hand (Fig. 56).

5. With the arms straight, rock forwards pressing down on the lower half of the breast-bone. (In an unconscious adult it can usually be pressed towards the spine for about one and a half inches (4 cm)).

In adults – repeat the pressure once per second:

In children the pressure of one hand is sufficient and the rate is 80–90 times per minute

For infants, use only light pressure with two fingers at the rate of 100 times per minute.

The pressure in all cases should be firm and controlled: *erratic or violent action may cause damage to the ribs or to internal organs.*

6. Check the effectiveness of the compression of the heart by –

– watching for an improvement in the casualty's colour;

– noting the size of the pupils, which should become smaller with effective treatment;

– feeling the carotid pulse, which should become apparent with each compression.

7. Emergency resuscitation may have to be continued until the casualty reaches hospital.

The rate of lung inflation and heart compression, based on present experience, is as follows –

One First Aider alone

Fifteen heart compressions followed by two quick lung inflations, and then repeat.

Two First Aiders

Five heart compressions followed by one deep lung inflation, and then repeat.

One First Aider should undertake the external heart compression, while the other First Aider undertakes the inflation, noting the size of the pupils and feeling for the carotid pulse.

Holger Nielsen method of artificial respiration

If ventilation of the lungs by the mouth-to-mouth (mouth-to-nose) method cannot be undertaken because of severe facial injuries, or when the casualty is trapped in the face-downwards position, the Holger Nielsen method is recommended. It is not practicable when there are gross injuries to the upper limbs, shoulder-girdle or ribs.

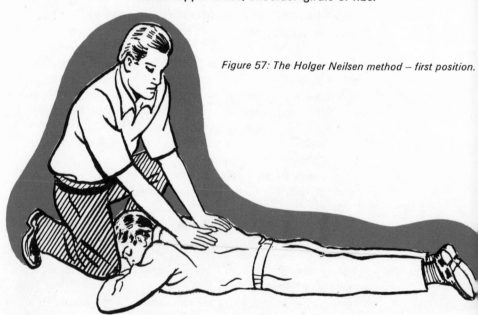

Figure 57: The Holger Neilsen method – first position.

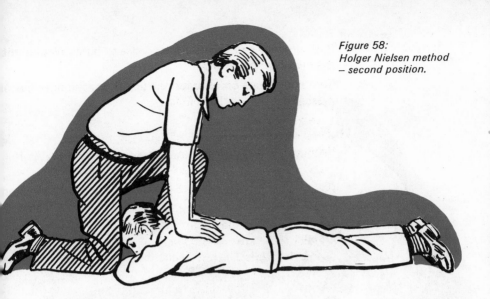

Figure 58:
Holger Nielsen method
– second position.

Position of casualty

1. The casualty should be placed faced downwards on a flat surface.

2. His hands, one over the other, should be placed level with his forehead, the casualty's head being turned to one side so that his cheek rests on the uppermost hand.

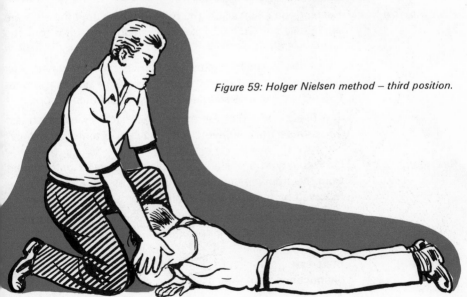

Figure 59: Holger Nielsen method – third position.

Position of the operator

Kneel on one knee at casualty's head, and put the foot of the other leg near his elbow.

Place your hands on his back just below the shoulder-blade.

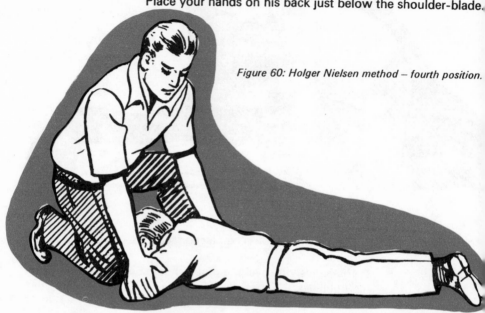

Figure 60: Holger Nielsen method – fourth position.

Application

Keeping the elbows straight, rock forwards until the arms are approximately vertical, exerting steady pressure on the casualty's chest.

Grasp the casualty's arms just above the elbow and rock backwards, raising his arms until resistance and tension are felt at the casualty's shoulders. The arms are then dropped.

The phases of expansion and compression should each last $2\frac{1}{2}$ seconds, the complete cycle repeated 12 times per minute.

Recovery

On recovery at any stage, outpouring of saliva and of fluid from the stomach and nose usually takes place: this may be followed by retching and vomiting.

To prevent inhalation of this fluid or vomit, place the casualty carefully in the recovery position.

Special treatment

Drowning

Start resuscitation immediately, quickly removing any obvious obstructions from the casualty's mouth.

Arrange for urgent removal to hospital.

54

Suffocation by poisonous gases

The use of a *life-line* when entering a gas filled room or space is a safety precaution and should be used wherever possible.

1. Before entering the area breathe in and out several times and then take a deep breath and hold it.

2. Go in and remove the casualty to safety.

3. If breathing is failing or has stopped, start resuscitation immediately.

Note. If it is not possible to rescue the casualty at once, **endeavour to cut off the source of danger** – turn off the gas, switch off the engine, and obtain a full supply of fresh air by opening doors and windows.

Suffocation by smoke

Protect yourself from loose carbon particles by tying a towel or coarse cloth, preferably wet, over your mouth and nose.

Keep low and remove the casualty as quickly as possible.

The use of a *life-line* is a valuable safety precaution and should be used wherever possible.

Choking

A common incident at all ages. Although a foreign body may be present, the obstruction to breathing is largely due to spasm.

Signs and symptoms

The casualty may have a fit of coughing; his face and neck are congested and may become livid. Violent and alarming attempts at inspiration may be made.

Treatment

The aim of first aid is to remove any foreign body and relieve the spasm, and, if necessary, to get air into the lungs past the foreign body.

Remove any obvious obstruction. If the obstruction is thought to be in the windpipe, in the case of:

An infant –
1. Hold the infant up by his legs.
2. Smack him smartly three or four times between the shoulders (Fig. 61).

A child –
1. Lay the child over your knee, head dowards.
2. Give three or four sharp slaps between the shoulders (Fig. 62).

55

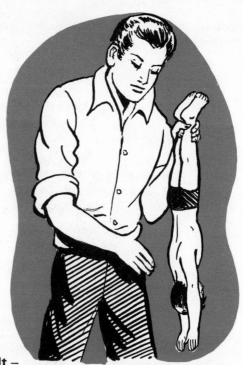

Figure 61:
Removing an obstruction from the windpipe of an infant.

An adult –

1. Immediately strike the adult three or four sharp blows between the shoulders.

In all cases, after clearing any obstruction from the throat, give artificial respiration, if necessary.

Hanging, strangulation, throttling

1. Remove the cause or relieve the obstruction –
– tear open the plastic bag;
– cut and remove any obstruction round the throat, supporting the weight of the body in cases of hanging;
2. Give artificial respiration, if necessary.

Electrical injuries
Low voltage (domestic supply)

Even with domestic voltages if an electric current passes through a person it may, in some cases, produce irregular quivering or tremor of muscles of the heart or stop its action with cessation of breathing. Burns may also be present.

Action

1. Break the contact – switch off the current, remove the plug or wrench the cable free.
2. If it is not possible to switch off or break the current, the

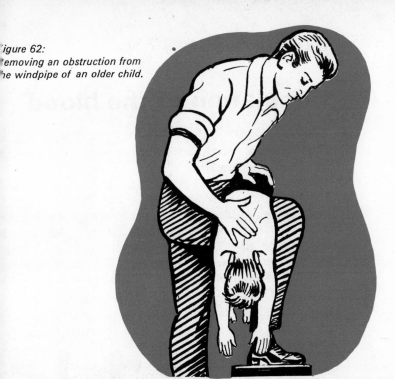

Figure 62:
Removing an obstruction from
the windpipe of an older child.

casualty must be removed from contact with it. Before attempting to do this, ensure that you are properly insulated otherwise you may also be affected.

3. With ordinary domestic voltages, insulation can be obtained by wearing rubber gloves or by standing on a rubber surface or thick layers of dry cloth or newspapers.

4. Withdraw the casualty by grasping dry clothing or by pulling him away with a dry rope or walking stick. Avoid anything damp or metallic.

5. **If breathing is absent, commence artificial respiration immediately.**

6. Treat burns, if present.

High voltage injuries

Do not attempt to rescue.
No safe approach to render first aid can be made.
Keep all persons back by at least twenty yards.
Get someone to contact the police.

CHAPTER FIVE •

Circulation of the blood

The circulatory system consists of the *heart*, the *arteries*, th[
capillaries and the *veins*.

The heart

The **heart** is a muscular organ which acts like a doubl[
pump. It lies in the chest cavity between the two lung[
It is divided into a right and left side, and each side is furthe[
divided into an upper collecting chamber (*atrium*) and [
lower pumping chamber (*ventricle*). The circulation is con[
trolled between these chambers by non-return valves.

The heart beats at approximately 72 times per minute in a[
adult at rest, but is faster in children (approximately 100 time[
per minute), also in exercise, fever, emotional stress an[
after the consumption of alcohol.

*Figure 63: Diagram of the heart
and great vessels.*

The valves are:
1. *Atrio-ventricular (right).*
2. *Pulmonary (right).*
3. *Atrio-ventricular (left).*
4. *Aortic (left).*

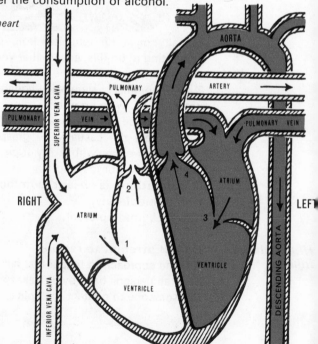

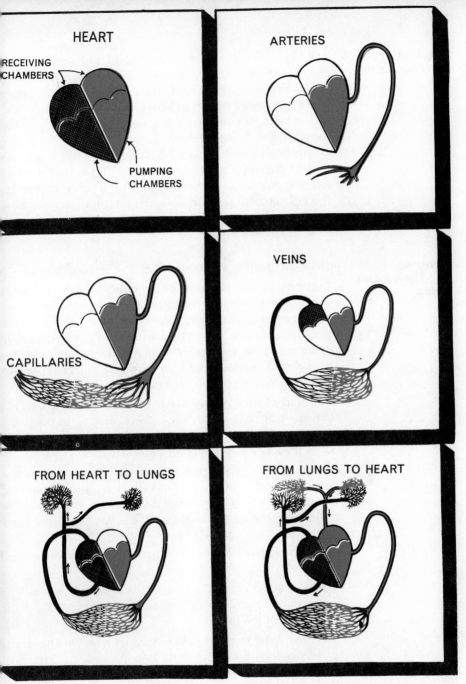

Figure 64: Circulation of the blood

With acknowledgments to First Aid Training Wing, R.A.M.C.

Mechanism of the circulation

The right ventricle pumps the blood through the lung (*pulmonary circulation*) and the left ventricle pumps th fresh blood through the body (*systemic circulation*). Venou blood is collected from the upper and lower parts of the bod in the right atrium where it passes through to the righ ventricle and is then forced through arteries to the lung where it gives off its impurities, carbon dioxide gas, an obtains oxygen from the inspired air. This blood, rich wit oxygen, returns to the left atrium of the heart, passes int the left ventricle when it is forced out into the main arter (*aorta*), and then through its many branches is distributed t all parts of the body.

Arteries, capillaries and veins

These are the tubes through which the blood circulates.

Arteries are the strongest of the blood vessels, their wall being strengthened by elastic and muscular tissue with fibrous covering, and they carry blood away from the hear They expand with the volume of blood forced along then by the pumping action of the heart and then return to thei normal size. Arteries continue to divide becoming smalle and smaller until they become capillaries.

Capillaries are very small blood vessels, consisting only of thin layer of cells which allow the exchange of fluids anc gases to and from the tissue cells of the body. The tiny capil- laries gradually join up and become veins.

Veins, small at first, gradually becoming larger and large until they end in two large veins which returns the blood to the right collecting chamber of the heart. Veins have cuplike valves which allow the blood to flow only towards the heart

The pulse

The pulse is the pressure wave indicating the contraction o the heart.

It is normally taken at the front of the wrist, where it can be felt about half-an-inch (1 cm) from the thumb side of the lower end of the forearm.

The First Aider must be able to take its rate, whether faster or slower than normal, and its strength, whether strong or feeble. It may occasionally be irregular. Make a note of your findings and the time it was taken: these may be of great assistance subsequently to a doctor or hospital.

60

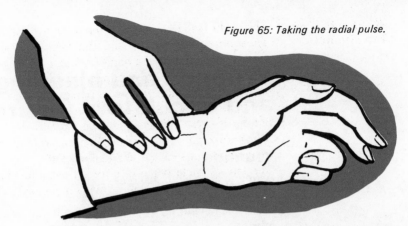

Figure 65: Taking the radial pulse.

Blood

Blood is the liquid which flows in the blood vessels, and consists of a transparent yellow fluid called blood *plasma* in which are suspended large numbers of *red and white blood cells* and blood *platelets.* There are many more red cells than white, hence the colour given to the blood. The colouring pigment in the red cells is called *haemoglobin*, which is the main carrier of oxygen to the tissue cells and accounts for the bright red colour of blood when oxygen is present, and the darker colour when oxygen is absent. The red cells are circular in shape and are hollowed out on either side. White blood cells are more irregular in shape, their duty being to engulf and remove harmful bodies in the tissues, such as dead bacteria and cells. As well as carrying oxygen to the tissue cells, the blood carries nutritive matter from the organs of digestion and also removes waste products, carrying them to the excretory organs, the lungs, kidneys and the skin.

Blood volume

The total quantity of blood circulating in the body of an average adult is about 10 to 11 pints (approximately 6 litres) or roughly a pint per stone of body weight. When much blood is lost from the circulation, the vital organs are deprived of fresh supplies of oxygen and nutritive matter, and shock develops.

Clotting of blood

When blood escapes from a damaged blood vessel it normally forms a clot. This is due to the formation of threads of fibrin in the plasma, which hold the blood platelets together in a fine mesh. Clotting is a valuable help in the stopping of bleeding, and in the prevention of infection into a wound. Clots in a wound should never be disturbed.

61

CHAPTER SIX

Wounds and bleeding and circulatory failure

Wounds

A wound is an abnormal break in the continuity of the tissues of the body which permits the escape of blood, externally or internally, and may allow the entrance of germs, causing infection.

Wounds may be classified as —
1. Incised or clean cut;
2. Lacerated or torn;
3. Contused or bruised;
4. Punctured or stab;
5. Gunshot, which may have a small entry but a large exit wound.

Bleeding

Bleeding may occur externally or internally and may vary from trivial to severe or fatal.

The body possesses certain in-built mechanisms that tend to stop bleeding spontaneously, and it is important to realise this. For example —

(a) Shed blood tends to clot so blocking the damaged vessels.

(b) The cut ends of the blood vessel, especially an artery, will contract thus lessening the loss of blood.

(c) The blood pressure will fall and consequently less blood is pushed out of the vessel.

External bleeding

Wounds with slight bleeding

Blood may ooze from all parts of the wound and may appear alarming, but the bleeding usually stops of its own accord. It is easily controlled by local pressure.

Treatment

1. Apply firm pressure to the bleeding points over a sterile

dressing, and bandage with a pad if necessary. An adhesive dressing may be sufficient.

2. Elevate the bleeding part and support in position, unless an underlying fracture is suspected.

3. Before applying the dressing, if the wound is dirty wash it with running water from the centre outwards, if possible. Protect with a sterile swab and gently clean the surrounding skin.

4. Dry the skin with swabs of cotton wool, using each swab once only, wiping away from the wound.

Wounds with severe bleeding

Severe bleeding may create a serious condition in which life is endangered.

Treatment

The aim of First Aid is to stop the bleeding immediately and to obtain medical aid urgently.

1. Apply direct pressure with the fingers to the bleeding point or points, over a dressing if available, for 5–15 minutes. If the wound area is large, press the sides of the wound firmly but gently together.

2. Lay the casualty down in a suitable and comfortable position, and lower the head if possible.

3. Raise the injured part and support in position, unless an underlying fracture is suspected.

4. Carefully remove from the wound any foreign bodies which are visible and can easily be picked out or wiped off with a dressing.

5. Apply a sterile dressing to the wound and press it firmly down into the wound, cover it with a pad of soft material and retain the dressing and pad in position with a firm bandage. Ensure that the dressing and pad extend well above the level and well beyond the edges of the wound.

6. If bleeding continues, apply further dressings and pads on top of the original dressing, and bandage more firmly.

7. Immobilise the injured part by a suitable method, e.g. a sling for the upper limb, or tying an uninjured lower limb to an injured one.

8. Remove to hospital as soon as possible.

Foreign bodies in wound

When it is not possible to remove a foreign body or if the ends of a broken bone protrude through the skin –

1. Apply pressure alongside the wound, or press the side of the wound firmly but gently together.

2. Apply a dressing to the wound.

3. Place pads of cotton wool or other soft material round the wound to a sufficient height to prevent pressure on the foreign body. A ring pad may be used.

4. Secure the dressing and pads with a bandage applied diagonally, thus avoiding the danger of pressure on the foreign body.

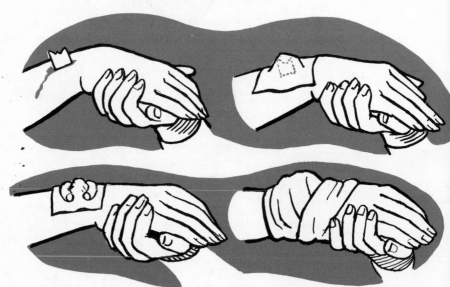

Figure 66: Treatment of a wound with object embedded in flesh.

Indirect pressure

If bleeding cannot be controlled by the application of direct pressure on the wound or when it is impossible to apply direct pressure successfully, it may be possible to apply indirect pressure at the appropriate pressure point between the heart and the wound.

A pressure point is where an important artery can be compressed against an underlying bone to prevent the flow of blood beyond that point. Such pressure may be applied while dressing, pad and bandage are being prepared for application, but not for longer than 15 minutes at a time.

Brachial pressure point

The brachial artery runs along the inner side of the muscle of the upper arm, its course being roughly indicated by the inner seam of a coat sleeve.

To apply pressure, pass your fingers under the casualty's upper arm and compress the artery against the bone (*humerus*) (Fig. 67).

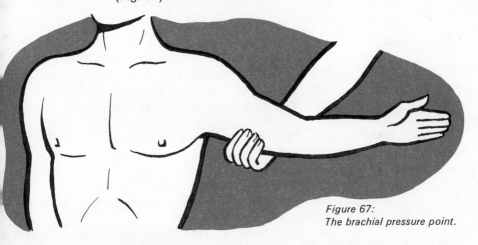

Figure 67:
The brachial pressure point.

Femoral pressure point

The femoral artery passes into the lower limb at a point corresponding to the fold of the groin.

To apply pressure, bend the casualty's knee, grasp his thigh with both hands and press directly and firmly downwards in the centre of the groin with both thumbs, one on top of the other, against the brim of the pelvis (Fig. 68).

Figure 68:
The femoral pressure point.

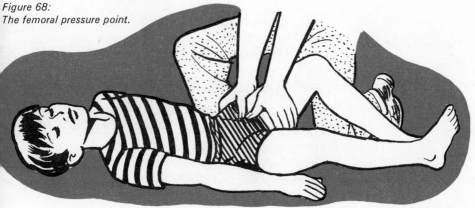

Internal bleeding Internal bleeding may occur following a broken bone, or result from a blow or bullet, a stab wound or a crush injury. It may also be associated with certain medical conditions in which there are no discernible causes.

Internal bleeding may –
– remain concealed;
– subsequently become visible.

Concealed Bleeding may remain concealed in the following cases –
– fracture of the vault of the skull, or cerebral bleeding;
– bleeding into the tissues, associated with fractures;
– from the spleen, liver or other organs into the abdomen. This source of bleeding can be very dangerous.

Subsequently visible Internal bleeding may become visible in the following ways –
– when blood issues from the ear canal or nose or appears as a bloodshot eye, or is swallowed and afterwards vomited, as in the case of a fractured base of the skull;
– from the lungs when blood, bright red and frothy, is coughed up;
– from the stomach when blood is vomited. If vomited immediately, this blood will be bright red: if it has remained in the stomach for some time, it will resemble coffee grounds;
– from the upper bowel, when partly digested blood is passed in the motions, giving them a black tarry appearance;
– from the lower bowel, when blood normal in appearance, is passed in the motions;
– from the kidneys or bladder, when blood escaping into the urine may make it smoky or red in appearance.

Treatment (concealed or visible) **The aim of First Aid is to obtain medical aid immediately, and to combat shock (see page 75).**
1. Place the casualty at complete rest with legs raised; warn him not to move.
2. Loosen all tight clothing about his neck, chest and waist.
3. Reassure him and explain the necessity to relax mentally and physically.
4. Examine for any other injuries: the casualty's word may not be reliable in severe cases.
5. Protect him from cold.
6. Remove to hospital immediately in as quiet and gentle a manner as possible.

7. Keep careful watch on his breathing and pulse rate. Make a written note of the pulse and time of recording for the doctor. If removal to hospital is delayed, record pulse rate at 10–15 minute intervals.

8. Keep record of any specimen passed or vomited.

Do not give anything by the mouth.

Blood loss

Signs and symptoms

As the result of severe loss of blood, *external or internal*, the following occurs –

– Face and lips become pale.
– Skin is cold and clammy.
– Casualty feels faint and dizzy.
– Pulse is rapid, becoming weaker.
– Restlessness: casualty complains of thirst.
– Breathing becomes shallow, sometimes accompanied by yawning and sighing; casualty may gasp for air ('air hunger.')

These signs and symptoms may vary widely in different persons and in different circumstances and with the rate of bleeding.

Bleeding from special areas

From the scalp

Wounds of the scalp may cause severe and alarming bleeding.

Treatment

Do not press into or probe the wound – there may be an underlying fracture.

1. Apply a dressing much larger than the wound and bandage firmly in position.

2. If an underlying fracture is suspected or there is a foreign body in the wound, a large ring pad should be used to permit pressure around the wound but not on the fracture or foreign body.

3. Refer casualty quickly to hospital for further treatment.

From the ear canal

Bleeding or perhaps discharge of straw-coloured fluid from the ear canal may indicate a fracture of the base of the skull (see page 82).

Treatment

1. Place a dressing or pad over the ear and secure lightly in position.

2. Lay the casualty down with the head slightly raised and inclined to the injured side, or if unconscious in the recovery position.

3. Remove to hospital immediately.

4. Keep careful watch on his breathing and pulse rate.

From the nose
Treatment

1. Support the casualty in a sitting position with his head slightly forward.

2. Instruct him to breathe through his mouth.

3. Pinch the soft part of the nose firmly for about 10 minutes.

4. Loosen clothing about the neck and chest.

5. Warn him not to blow his nose.

If bleeding does not stop within a short time, or recurs, the casualty should receive medical attention.

From a tooth socket (gums)
Treatment

1. Place a pad of cotton wool or gauze firmly in the socket. This pad must be large enough to prevent the teeth meeting when the pad is bitten on.

2. Instruct the casualty to bite on the pad for 10 to 20 minutes.

If bleeding is not controlled seek dental or medical advice. *Do not* wash out the mouth, as this may disturb clotting. *Do not* plug the socket.

From the tongue or cheek

Compress the part between the finger and thumb, using a clean handkerchief or dressing, if available.

From the palm of the hand

Bleeding may be severe as several blood vessels may be involved.

Treatment

1. Apply direct pressure.

2. Raise the limb if no fracture is suspected.

When no fracture or removable foreign body is present
1. Cover the wound with a dressing and place a suitable pad over it.

2. Bend the fingers over the pad so as to make a fist.

3. Bandage the fingers firmly with a folded triangular bandage; tying off across the knuckles.

4. Support the limb in a triangular sling.

When there is a fracture or irremovable foreign body present
1. Treat the wound.

2. Support in a triangular sling.

Chest injuries

Penetrating (stab) wound of the chest

A wound in the chest wall may allow direct access of air into the chest cavity. During *inspiration*, the noise of air being sucked in may be heard; on *expiration* blood or blood-stained bubbles may be expelled from the wound.

If the lung is injured, the casualty may also cough up frothy bright red blood.

Treatment

The aim of First Aid is to seal the wound immediately and to stop air entering the chest cavity.
1. Until a dressing can be applied, place the palm of the hand firmly over the wound.
2. Lay the casualty down with head and shoulders raised and the body inclined towards the injured side.
3. Plug the wound lightly with a dressing.
4. Cover the dressing with a thick layer of cotton wool.
5. Retain it firmly in position by strapping or a bandage.
6. *Remove to hospital urgently.*

Stove-in chest

An increasingly common example is the 'steering wheel' injury, caused when the driver of a motor vehicle is flung violently forward against the steering wheel. There may be a fracture of several ribs and of the breast-bone, parts of which may be driven inwards possibly damaging the heart, lungs or other internal organs.

Signs and symptoms

The casualty is severely distressed with difficultly in breathing. Blueness of the lips and extremities may be present.
The injured part of the chest wall will be seen to have lost its rigidity so that –
– during inspiration the injured part, instead of expanding with the chest, is sucked in, while
– on expiration, it is blown out.

Sufficient air does not enter the lungs and in consequence the blood cannot obtain enough oxygen.

Treatment

The aim of First Aid is to reduce respiratory activities to the minimum necessary.
1. Loosen any tight clothing – collar, belt, etc.
2. Place the casualty at rest.
3. Immobilise the injured part of the chest by placing the arm against it as a splint, but with the elbow bent.

4. Secure by strapping or bandaging the arm to the chest.
5. *Remove urgently to hospital.*

Raise the head of the stretcher to reduce pressure of the abdominal contents on the diaphragm.

Blast injuries

This injury is caused by an explosion.

The casualty may be apprehensive and in a tremulous state, and restless with pain in the chest. There may be blueness of the lips and extremities and frothy blood-stained sputum may be coughed up. Breathing may be difficult.

There may be no signs of bruising or of fractures, and, due to the shocked state, the casualty may not complain of pain or tenderness.

Treatment

1. Reassure the casualty, insisting that complete rest is essential.
2. Lay him down with head and shoulders raised and supported.
3. Loosen any tight clothing – collar, belt, etc.
4. *Remove urgently to hospital.*

Wounds of the abdominal wall

Treatment

Place the casualty so that the wound does not gape – preferably on his back with head and shoulders raised and supported with a pillow under his knees.

If no internal organs protrude –
Apply a dressing to the wound; bandage it firmly in position.

If internal organs protrude through the wound –
– cover them lightly with a soft clean towel or a large gauze dressing.
– secure without undue pressure.

In all cases –
– support the abdomen if vomiting or coughing is present;
– **remove urgently to hospital.**
Do not give anything by the mouth.

Varicose veins

Varicose veins occur when the valve of the veins, usually those of the legs, fail to act correctly. This is not commonly met with in the young. There is a back pressure and the veins enlarge forming a reservoir of blood.

Bleeding from a burst varicose vein in the leg may be *sudden, severe and spurting,* and if not immediately controlled may be fatal.

Treatment
1. Apply immediately direct pressure to the bleeding point, over a dressing if available.
2. Loosen any constriction such as a garter, which may impede circulation.
3. Lay the casualty flat on his back and raise the leg as high as possible.
4. Apply a dressing, pad and bandage firmly in position.
5. Keep the leg raised and supported.
6. Ensure that the casualty is seen by his own doctor or taken to hospital.

Bruises (contusion)

A bruise is bleeding beneath the unbroken skin often due to a fall or a blow on the surface of the body. The condition is a minor form of internal bleeding, but when extensive may have serious consequences.

The injury may be accompanied by pain, swelling and discoloration.

Treatment
1. Put the part at rest in the most comfortable position.
2. Apply a cold application as quickly as possible to reduce the swelling and to relieve pain.
Cold applications consist of –
– cold compress;
– ice bag.

Cold compress
(i) Soak a thin towel, large handkerchief, piece of flannel or absorbent cotton wool, in cold water;
(ii) squeeze out the surplus water and apply the compress to the bruised area;
(iii) keep it cool by dripping water on to it as required, or replace it by further compresses. Ensure good evaporation by not covering the compress, but if necessary, use open weave material to keep it in place.

Ice bag
(i) Fill a polythene (or non-porous) bag two-thirds full with crushed ice;

71

(ii) add some common salt to melt the ice and increase the cooling action;

(iii) expel the air and tie up the bag;

(iv) wrap the bag in a thin towel and apply it carefully to the bruised area;

(v) renew ice and salt as necessary.

Crush injury

This is a condition which may cause acute kidney failure especially if casualties have been crushed or trapped for more than an hour by some heavy weight such as masonry or machinery. Crush injuries involve soft tissues (muscles and skin) and sometimes fractures.

On release, the appearance of such casualties may be deceptive, showing little signs of injury except perhaps redness or swelling of the part. There may be some bruising or blister formation and casualties may complain of numbness and tingling.

Complications may occur some hours after release when the injured tissues may swell and become hard due to the outpouring of fluid (*plasma*) from the blood into them. Blood pressure falls and shock becomes more profound. Certain poisonous products of the injured muscles are absorbed into the bloodstream and can lead to acute kidney failure and death.

Treatment

1. On release, keep the casualty on his back with head low and lower limbs raised, if possible. Warn him not to move.

2. Arrange for removal to hospital with the least delay, as this is the danger period. It is important to inform the hospital of the possibility of crush injury as initially there may be little evidence of it.

3. If conscious and an internal abdominal injury is not suspected, give an adult casualty sips of water to wash out his mouth, otherwise *no fluid* is to be given as he may require an anaesthetic on admission to hospital. Record quantity of fluid given.

4. Reassure the casualty.

5. Leave an injured limb uncovered.

Acute heart attacks

These result from a reduction of blood supply to the muscular wall of the heart. There are two varieties:

Angina pectoris Where the arteries to the heart have become too narrow for an adequate supply of blood to the heart muscle. Excitement or over exertion brings on an attack of pain in the chest which often spreads to the left shoulder and arm and to the fingers. The pain may also spread to the throat and jaws and even to the other upper limb.

Coronary obstruction Where the blood clots suddenly in a coronary artery in the wall of the heart and blocks it. The casualty is gripped by an excruciating vice-like pain behind the breast-bone, which may spread into the upper limbs, throat and jaw.

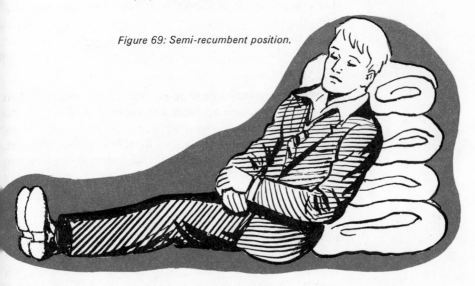

Figure 69: Semi-recumbent position.

Signs and symptoms

In both cases the casualty –
– suffers from severe pain and shock which may force him to stop what he is doing. He sits down or leans against a wall for support;
– he may also feel giddy and sink to the ground;
– he is often short of breath;
– he may become unconscious.
– the pulse is weak and may become irregular.

73

Treatment

The aim of First Aid is to reduce the work of the heart and sustain the casualty during an attack.

1. *Do not* move the casualty unnecessarily but place him in the most comfortable position which is usually –

– semi-recumbent with his head and shoulders raised on two or more pillows, *or*

– supported in a sitting position if this makes his breathing easier.

2. Loosen clothing about the neck, chest and waist.

3. If breathing fails begin artificial respiration immediately and if necessary, give external heart compression. Both these procedures may have to be continued on the way to hospital.

4. *Arrange for urgent transport to hospital,* obtaining medical aid if available.

The casualty may require the administration of oxygen.

Note. People liable to angina pectoris often carry tablets (glyceryl trinitrate). *Do not* administer these tablets to the casualty as they are not useful in the treatment of a case but only for the prevention of an attack.

In other suspected heart cases
Treat as for Acute Heart attack, *except* –
Place the casualty in a sitting position.
Do not lay him flat as he will not be able to get sufficient air into his lungs and he may become asphyxiated.

CHAPTER SEVEN

Shock

Shock is a condition arising from stress or injury causing an insufficient supply of blood to the brain, which causes a lessening of activities and affects the vital functions of the body. It may accompany injuries, bleeding, severe pain or sudden illness. The severity of shock depends upon the nature and extent of the injury or other causes and may vary from a feeling of faintness even unto sudden death.

Causes

Severe bleeding – either external or internal.
Loss of Plasma – in burns or crush injuries.
Heart failure – as in acute heart attacks.

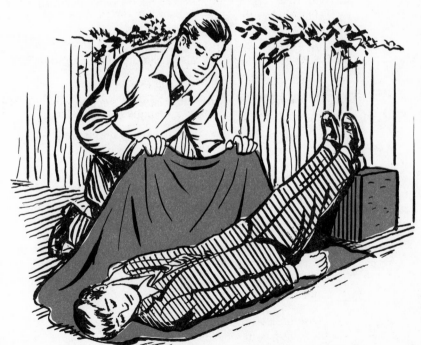

Figure 70: Protect shock casualty from contact with the bare ground by using a blanket or something similar.

Acute abdominal emergencies – perforation of stomach ruptured appendix.

Loss of body fluid – recurrent vomiting from any cause or severe diarrhoea.

Nerve stimulation – nerve shock caused by sensory nerve stimulation usually but not always painful.

Signs and symptoms

Casualty will become extremely pale;
– his skin will be cold and clammy with profuse sweating;
– he may feel faint and giddy or sick and may vomit;
– he may complain of thirst and feel anxious;
– his pulse increases in rate tending to become weak and thready;
– breathing is shallow and rapid;
– consciousness may be clouded.

Treatment

1. Lay the casualty down and deal with the injury or underlying cause of the shock.

2. Keep his head low and turned to one side, raise the lower limbs when possible.

If there is an injury to his head, chest or abdomen, the shoulders should be raised slightly and supported, with his head turned to one side;

If vomiting seems likely or if he is unconscious, place him carefully in the recovery position.

3. Loosen clothing at the neck, chest and waist.

4. If casualty complains of thirst, moisten his lips with water.

5. Protect if necessary with a blanket or sheet.

6. Keep frequent records of the pulse and respiration rates if removal to hospital is likely to be delayed.

When the condition of the casualty clearly indicates hospital or medical attention, *do not* waste valuable time by over-elaborate first aid measures, but get him to hospital as quickly as possible.

Do not use hot water bottles.
Do not give the casualty anything to drink.
Do not move him unnecessarily. The more serious the injury, the more important it is **not** to move the casualty.

Fainting

Fainting follows a temporary reduction in blood supply to the brain. It may begin with a feeling of faintness and lead to a collapse. Some degree of nerve shock accompanies all injuries.

Causes

Emotional or sensory stimulus –
– a fright, bad news, a horrifying sight, or pain;
– fatigue, long periods of sitting or standing in a hot stuffy atmosphere;
– a debilitating illness *or*
– injury to some part of the body.

Impending faint

There may be some warning before fainting – the person may yawn or sway and feel unsteady and become giddy, his face becomes pale or greenish-white, beads of sweat are

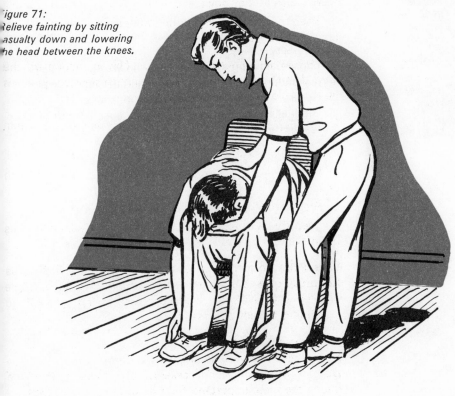

*Figure 71:
Relieve fainting by sitting casualty down and lowering the head between the knees.*

seen on his face, neck and hands, and his consciousness is clouded.

If this occurs –

1. Reassure the casualty and urge him to breathe deeply.
2. Loosen clothing at neck, chest and waist.
3. Lay him down in a current of fresh air, or sit him down and lower his head between his knees.
4. On recovery, sips of water may be given.
5. Smelling salts may be useful: test their strength before use.

Signs and symptoms of a faint

The casualty is unconscious –
– his face is pale with skin cold and clammy;
– breathing is shallow;
– pulse is weak and slow at first but gradually increases in rate.

Treatment of a faint

1. Lay the casualty down and deal with any cause. If possible raise the legs slightly above the level of the head.
2. See that he has plenty of fresh air; place him in the shade if necessary.
3. Loosen clothing at neck, chest and waist.
4. If breathing is difficult, place him in the recovery position.
5. Reassure him as he regains consciousness.
6. Gradually raise him into the sitting position and give sips of water, if required.

CHAPTER EIGHT

Injuries to bones

Fractures

A broken or cracked bone is described as a fracture. When a diagnosis is uncertain treat all such injuries as fractures.

Causes

Direct Force –
– when the bone breaks at the spot where the force is applied, e.g. from a kick or blow.

Indirect Force –
(a) when the bone breaks at some distance from the spot where the force is applied, e.g. a fall on the outstretched hand, which may cause a fracture of the collar-bone;
(b) when there is a sudden violent contraction of the muscles which may cause a fracture, e.g. the knee-cap.

Types of fracture

Closed – when the surface of the skin is not broken (Fig. 72).

Figure 72:
Closed fracture.

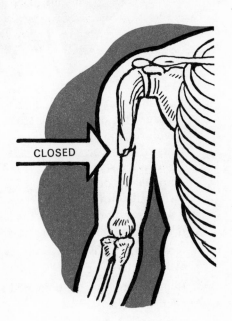

CLOSED

Open – when there is a wound leading down to the fracture or when the fractured ends protrude through the skin, thus allowing germs to gain access to the soft tissues and broken bone (Fig. 73).

When there is associated injury to an important structure such as the brain, major blood vessels, nerves, lungs, liver or when associated with a dislocation of a joint, either type of fracture is said to be *complicated* (Fig. 74).

Figure 73:
Open fracture.

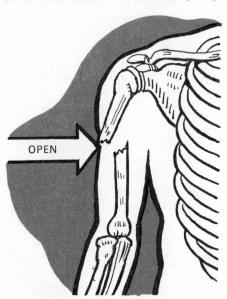

OPEN

Signs and symptoms

Pain in or near the injured part.
Tenderness on gentle pressure.
Swelling and later bruising.
Loss of control.
Deformity such as –
– irregularity of the bone;
– shortening of the limb;
– angulation or rotation of the limb;
– depression of a flat bone.

Not all the above signs and symptoms may be present in every fracture.

Comparison with the uninjured side will often help in the diagnosis.

80

Figure 74:
Complicated fracture.

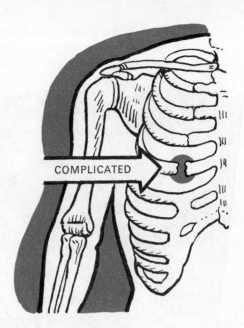

COMPLICATED

General rules for treatment

1. Asphyxia, bleeding and severe wounds must be dealt with before treating any fracture.

2. Treat the fracture where the casualty lies. The injured part must be secured, even if only in a temporary way, before the casualty is moved, unless life is immediately in danger.

3. Steady and support the injured part at once and maintain this control until the fracture is completely secured.

4. Immobilise the fracture by securing the injured part to a sound part of the body by means of bandages, or where necessary, by the use of splints and bandages.

Using bandages alone

Bandages should be applied sufficiently firmly to prevent movement, but not so tightly as to interfere with the circulation of the blood or to cause pain.

To pass bandages under a casualty lying down, use the natural hollows of the body, e.g. the neck, loins, knees and ankles, and then gently work them into their correct position.

Using splints

Splints must be –
– well-padded and sufficiently rigid;
– long and wide enough to immobilise the joint above and below the fracture.

81

They may be improvised from a walking stick, umbrella, broom handle, piece of wood, cardboard or firmly folded newspaper or magazine. (Fig. 75).

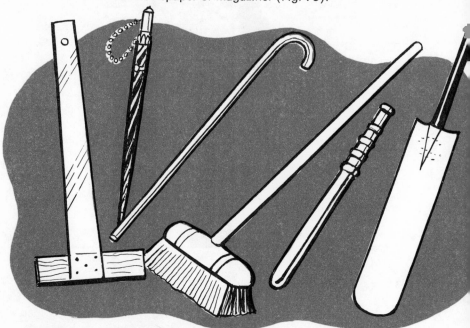

Figure 75: Useful items for improvised splints.

Special fractures

The skull

Fracture here is often complicated by some injury to the brain and may produce unconsciousness in varying degrees.

Fracture of the vault (cranium)
This is caused by a direct blow or fall on the head and the bone may be depressed inwards.

Fracture of the base
This is usually the result of indirect force – a severe blow on the lower jaw, or a fall on to the feet or lower part of the spine, transmitting the force to the base of the skull.

Signs and symptoms

Blood or straw-coloured fluid may issue from the ear canal or from the nose, or give the eye a bloodshot appearance and later a 'black-eye'.

Treatment

1. Place the casualty in the recovery position with adequate support.

2. Establish level of consciousness and check frequently.

3. If a discharge issues from the ear, turn the head so that the ear is downwards, and apply a sterile dressing and secure lightly.

4. Keep a careful watch on the casualty's breathing, ensure a clear airway, start artificial respiration if breathing stops or begins to fail.

5. Maintain casualty's position during transport and avoid unnecessary movement.

Fracture of the lower jaw

This is due to a direct blow on the jaw (Fig. 76). Usually only one side is affected. There may be a wound inside the mouth.

Special signs and symptoms

Pain, increased by jaw movements or by swallowing.
Difficulty in speaking.
Excessive flow of saliva, which is usually blood-stained.
Irregularity of the teeth.
Swelling, tenderness, and later bruising of the face and lower jaw.

Treatment

1. Maintain respiration by ensuring an open airway; ensure the tongue has not fallen to the back of the throat or that the mouth is not obstructed.

Figure 76: Fracture of the lower jaw by direct blow.

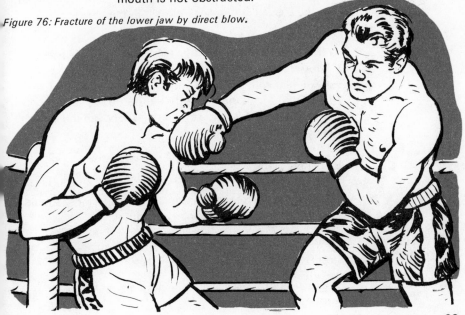

2. Control bleeding.

3. Remove any false teeth or broken loose teeth.

4. Support the jaw with a soft pad held in place by the hand or by a suitable bandage.

5. **If casualty conscious** – and not seriously injured –
– he may sit up with his head well forward to drain secretions.
If casualty unconscious –
– he must be placed in the recovery position, making sure that the jaw is kept well forward.

6. Support the jaw and head if vomiting occurs.

7. *Arrange urgent removal to hospital.*

Fracture of the spine

This is a grave and serious injury and may be caused by a fall of a heavy weight across the casualty's back or from impact in a vehicle, by a fall on the feet or buttocks, a fall on the head from a height as in diving, or over-flexion of the back muscles.

The fracture may be complicated by injury to the spinal cord causing loss of power and sensation in all parts of the body below the site of the fracture.

Fracture of the spine should always be suspected in all cases in which there is a history of injury to the vertebral column and the casualty complains of pain in the back.

Treatment

1. Immediately warn the casualty to lie still.

2. **If medical aid is readily available** –
– *Do not* move the casualty;
– cover him with a blanket and await the arrival of the doctor.
If medical aid is not readily available –
– carefully place pads of soft material between the casualty's thighs, knees and ankles;
– tie the ankles and feet together with a figure-of-eight bandage;
– apply broad bandages round the thighs and knees (Fig. 77).

The casualty, whether conscious or unconscious, should be transported in the face-upwards position.

Stretcher

Transport of a case of spinal injury

1. The canvas bed of a stretcher should be stiffened by placing boards across it.

2. Cover the boards with a folded blanket, then 'blanket the stretcher' (see page 137).

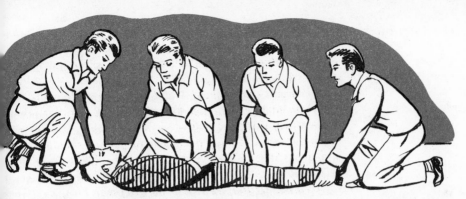

Figure 77: Fracture of the spine – preparation for transport.

3. Place pads on the stretcher to support the natural curves of the casualty's neck, small of back, knees and ankles.

Placing a blanket under casualty

When the casualty is not already lying on a blanket or rug and one is available –

1. Roll the blanket or rug lengthwise for half its width; place the roll in line with and against the casualty.

2. While two First Aiders maintain firm control of the head and lower limbs, the other First Aiders slowly and gently turn the casualty as in one piece on to his side, without bending the neck or twisting the trunk. Place the rolled portion of the blanket or rug close to the casualty's back and gently roll him over the roll until he is lying on his opposite side. The blanket or rug is then unrolled and the casualty gently turned on to his back. The two First Aiders controlling the head and lower limbs *must* maintain an even tension whilst the casualty is being turned and conform to the rolling of the casualty throughout (Fig. 78).

Figure 78: Rolling spinal casualty onto blanket.

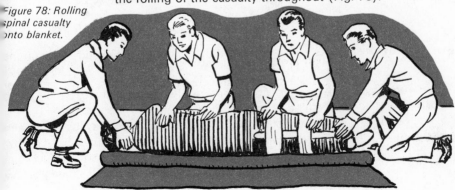

Loading the stretcher

1. Roll the two edges of the blanket up against the side of the casualty. If two stout poles of sufficient length are available, the edges of the blanket should be rolled round them. This makes lifting of the casualty easier.

2. While the two First Aiders continue to support the head and lower limbs, the remaining First Aiders place themselves on each side of the casualty facing one another. They carefully and evenly raise the casualty by grasping the rolled edges of the blanket to a sufficient height to enable the stretcher to be pushed under him. The casualty is then gently and cautiously lowered on to the stretcher. Ensure the pads on the stretcher are in the correct positions (Fig. 79).

In the case of a neck injury – place firm supports on each side of the head to steady it.

Figure 79: Placing spinal casualty on a stretcher.

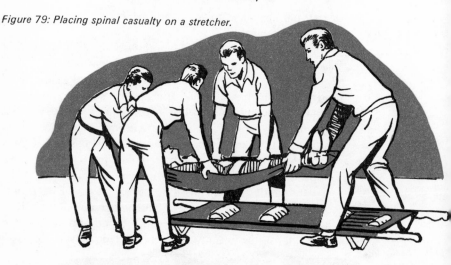

Fracture of the ribs

This is usually caused by a blow or by falling heavily on the chest (Fig. 80).

Signs and symptoms

Sharp pain at the site of the fracture, increased by deep breathing or coughing;

– If internal organs are affected, there may be signs and symptoms of internal bleeding;

– There may be an open wound of the chest wall over the fracture, causing a 'sucking wound' of the chest, which may allow direct access of air to the chest cavity.

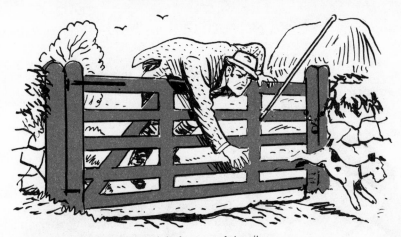

Figure 80: Situation which could result in fracture of the ribs.

Treatment

When the fracture is uncomplicated

1. Support the upper limb on the injured side in an arm sling.
2. Transport as a sitting or walking case unless otherwise indicated (Fig. 81).

When the fracture is complicated

1. A 'sucking wound' must be immediately treated (see page 69).

Figure 81: Treatment of an uncomplicated fracture of the ribs.

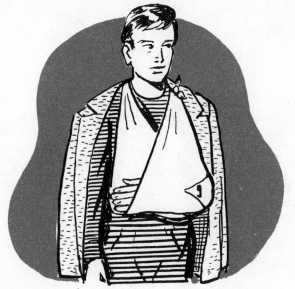

2. Support the upper limb on the injured side in a triangula
sling.

3. Lay the casualty down with head and shoulders raisec
and the body inclined towards the injured side. Support ir
this position by means of a folded blanket applied lengthwise
to his back (Fig. 82).

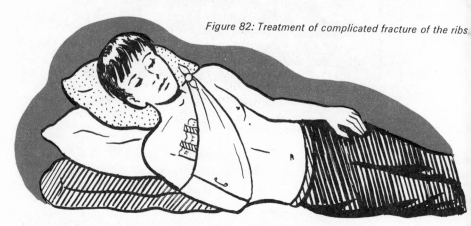

Figure 82: Treatment of complicated fracture of the ribs.

Fracture of the collar-bone

This is most commonly caused by a fall on the hand when the arm is outstretched from the side. (Fig. 83)

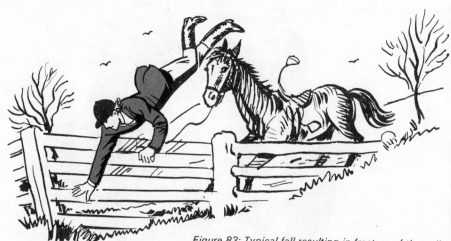

Figure 83: Typical fall resulting in fracture of the collar-bone.

88

Signs and symptoms	The arm on the injured side is partly helpless;
	– The casualty supports it at the elbow and keeps his head inclined towards the injured side;
	– Swelling or deformity can be seen or felt over the site of the fracture.
Treatment	1. Support the arm on the injured side.
	2. Pass a narrow bandage through each arm pit, encircle the shoulder and tie behind in a reef knot.
	3. Carry the free ends across the back over a pad placed between the shoulder-blades and tie the opposite ends together, or secure with a third bandage. As the knots are carefully tightened, the shoulders are braced well back in order to correct the overriding of the broken ends of the bone.
	4. Support the upper limb on the injured side in a triangular bandage. (Figs. 84, 85 and 86).

Fracture of the shoulder-blade

This is usually due to a blow or a crush.

Treatment

1. Remove overcoat and braces (if worn).
2. Place a pad in the armpit.
3. Support the upper limb on the injured side in a triangular sling.
4. Give further support by securing the upper limb to the chest by a broad bandage applied over the sling.

Fracture of the upper limb

This may take place anywhere along the bones of the limb and be near or even involve the elbow joint.

Treatment

Upper arm and forearm – if elbow is not involved

1. Place the forearm across the chest, fingers touching the fold of the opposite armpit.

2. Apply adequate soft padding between the limb and the chest.

3. Support the limb in an arm sling.

4. Give further support by securing the upper limb to the chest by a broad bandage applied over the sling.

5. Make sure pulse can still be felt at wrist.

If elbow cannot be bent without increasing pain

1. *Do not* attempt to force it.

2. Lay the casualty down and place the limb by his side, palm to thigh.

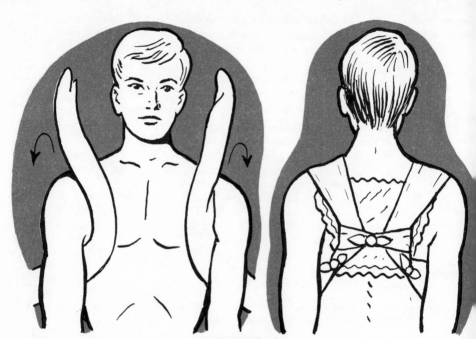

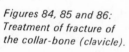

Figures 84, 85 and 86:
Treatment of fracture of
the collar-bone (clavicle).

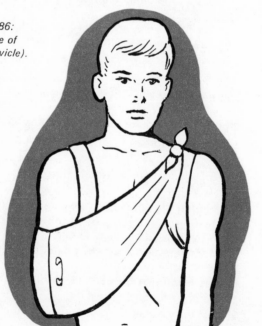

3. Apply adequate soft padding between the limb and the body.

4. Secure by three broad bandages, tied on the uninjured side of the body —

  (*i*) round the upper arm and trunk;

  (*ii*) round the forearm and trunk;

  (*iii*) round the wrist and thighs.

5. Transport as a stretcher case (Fig. 87).

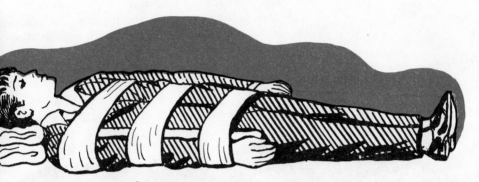

Figure 87: Treatment for fracture of the upper limb when elbow cannot be bent.

Wrist and lower end of forearm

1. Protect the forearm and wrist by placing it on a fold of soft padding.

2. Support the limb in an arm sling.

3. Give further support by securing the upper limb to the chest by a broad bandage applied over the sling.

Hand and Fingers

1. Protect the hand by placing it on a fold of soft padding.

2. Support the limb in a triangular sling.

3. Give further support by securing the upper limb to the chest by a broad bandage applied over the sling.

4. Make sure the pulse can still be felt at wrist.

Fracture of the pelvis

This is normally caused by a direct crush or by landing heavily on both feet. Pelvic organs, especially the bladder and urinary passages, may be injured.

Signs and symptoms

Pain in region of the hips and loins, increased by movement
— Inability to walk or stand;
— Urine may be passed and be coloured by blood;

91

Treatment

1. Lay the casualty in the position which gives the greatest comfort – usually on his back with his knees straight.
If he wishes to bend his knees slightly, they should be supported on a folded blanket.
2. Instruct casualty not to pass water.
3. **If journey to hospital is short and smooth –**
– transport as a stretcher case in the same position.

If journey to hospital is likely to be rough or there is some delay in reaching hospital –
(i) apply two broad bandages round the pelvis, overlapping by half, their centres in line with the hip joints of the affected side: tie off on the uninjured side;
(ii) place adequate soft padding between the knees and the ankles;
(iii) apply a figure-of-eight bandage round ankles and feet, and a broad bandage round the knees (Fig. 88).

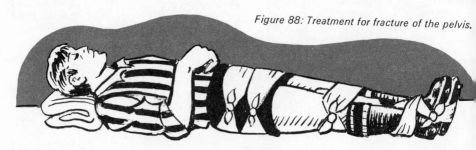

Figure 88: Treatment for fracture of the pelvis.

Fracture of the lower limb

The thigh bone may be broken anywhere along its length, but a fracture of the neck of the bone near the hip is very common in elderly people (Figs. 89 and 90).

Fractures of the thigh bone are always accompanied by severe shock.

The leg—One or both bones may be broken and usually a fracture of the tibia is open.

A fracture of the fibula two or three inches above the ankle (Pott's fracture) may be mistaken for a sprain of the ankle joint (Fig. 91).

Treatment

Fractures of major bones of the lower limb
1. Steady and support the injured limb.

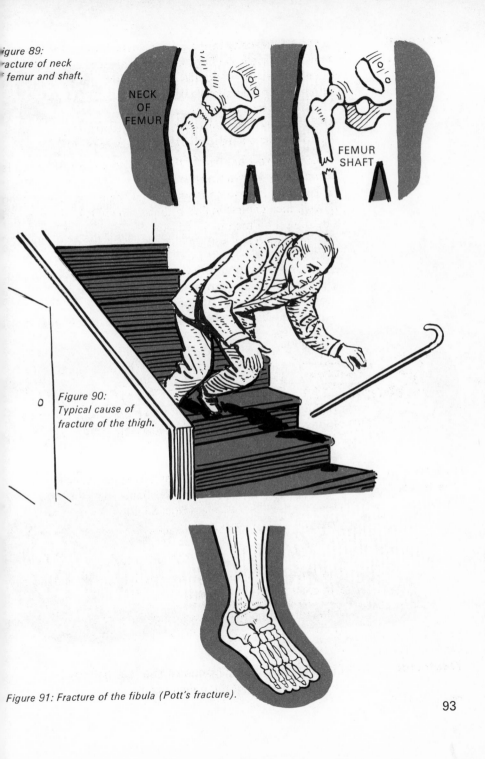

Figure 89:
Fracture of neck of femur and shaft.

NECK OF FEMUR

FEMUR SHAFT

Figure 90:
Typical cause of fracture of the thigh.

Figure 91: Fracture of the fibula (Pott's fracture).

93

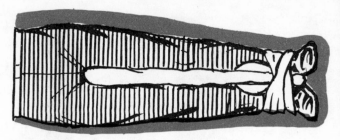

Figure 92: Use of a well-padded splint.

2. Bring the sound limb gently to the side of the injured one. If it is necessary to move the injured limb, gentle traction should be applied and maintained until the two limbs are tied together.

If journey to hospital is smooth and the casualty can be comfortably removed to hospital within half-an-hour of the arrival of the ambulance –
– place adequate soft padding between the thighs, knees and ankles;
– apply
(i) figure-of-eight bandage round the ankles and feet
(ii) broad bandage round the knees.

If journey to hospital is likely to be rough or long –
further secure by three broad bandages round –
(iii) the leg
(iv) the thighs
(v) below the site of the fracture ('floater bandage').

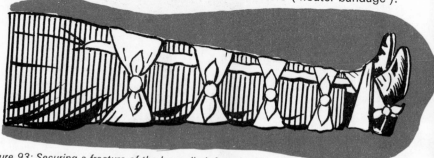

Figure 93: Securing a fracture of the lower limb for a long or rough journey.

Additionally a well-padded splint between the limbs extending from the crutch to the feet, may be used (Fig. 92).

1. Place a well-padded splint between the limbs, extending from the crutch to the feet, and an additional long padded splint to the side of the fractured limb, extending from the armpit to the foot.

2. Apply seven bandages in the following order –
  (i) the chest, just below the armpits
  (ii) the pelvis, in line with the hip joints
  (iii) ankles and feet
  (iv) the thighs, where possible above the fracture
  (v) the thighs, below the fracture ('floater bandage')
  (vi) the knees
  (vii) the legs
(Fig. 94).

In some instances one bandage may have to be omitted in order to avoid pressure over the site of the fracture.

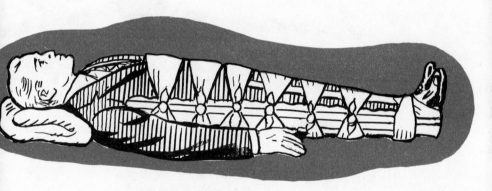

Figure 94: Treatment of fracture of the thigh.

Fracture of the knee-cap

This may be caused by muscular action which causes the bone to snap in two, or by direct force (Fig. 95).

Treatment

1. Lay the casualty on his back with head and shoulders raised and supported and the injured limb raised to a comfortable position and supported.

2. Apply a splint along the back of the limb, reaching from the crutch to beyond the heel, with adequate soft padding under the knee and also under the heel to raise it from the splint.

3. Secure the splint by three bandages –
   (*i*) figure-of-eight round ankle and foot
   (*ii*) broad bandage round the thigh
   (*iii*) broad bandage round the lower leg.

4. Keep the injured limb supported in a raised position (Fig. 96).

Fracture of the foot

This injury is usually caused by a heavy weight dropping on it, or a vehicle going over the foot (Fig. 97).

Treatment

1. Carefully remove footwear and sock or stocking, cutting if necessary.

2. Treat a wound, if present.

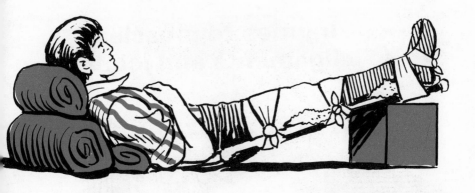

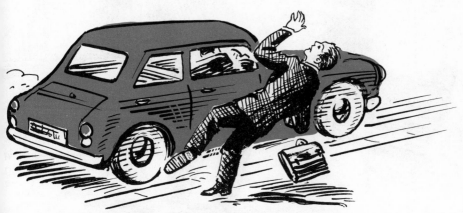

*Figure 97: A vehicle running over the foot may cause a
fracture.*

3. Apply a well-padded splint to the sole of the foot, reaching from the heel to the toes.

4. Secure the splint with a figure-of-eight bandage as follows –

place the centre of a broad bandage on the splint, cross the ends over the instep, carry them to the back of the ankle, cross them once more and pass them under the sole of the foot and tie off over the splint.

5. Raise and support the foot in a comfortable position.

All casualties with fractures of the lower limbs must be transported by stretcher.

97

CHAPTER NINE

Injuries to muscles, ligaments and joints

Strain

A strain is the over-stretching of a muscle (Fig. 98).

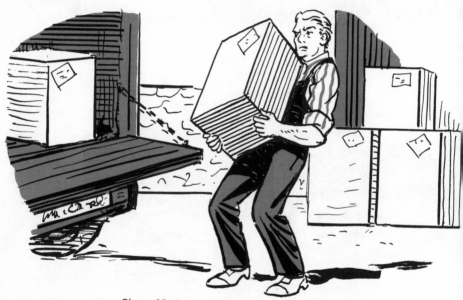

Figure 98: A common cause of strain.

Signs and symptoms	Sudden sharp pain at the site of the injury. In the case of a limb, the muscle may swell and cause severe cramp.
Treatment	Place the casualty in the most comfortable position, steady and support the injured part, arrange for medical aid.

Sprain

A sprain occurs at a joint where there is wrenching or tearing of the ligaments and tissues.

Pain at the joint;
– Swelling and later bruising;
– Inability to use the joint without increasing the pain.

1. Support the joint in the most comfortable position.
2. Carefully expose the joint and apply a firm bandage over a good layer of cotton wool, or apply a cold compress.

When a sprain of an ankle occurs out-of-doors, *do not* remove the boot or shoe but give additional support by applying a figure-of-eight bandage over the boot or shoe.

Dislocation

A dislocation is the displacement of one or more bones at a joint: it usually occurs in the shoulder, elbow, thumb, fingers and the lower jaw (Fig. 99).

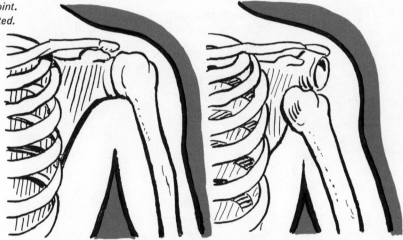

Pain, severe and sickening in character, near the joint;
– Fixity of the joint – casualty cannot move it;
– Deformity – abnormal appearance;
– Swelling and bruising are usually present.

1. Support and secure the part in the most comfortable position using pillows, cushions or bandages and slings.
2. Obtain medical aid at once.

Do not attempt to replace the bones to a normal position.

A dislocation may be complicated by the presence of a fracture. In any case of doubt, treat as for a fracture.

Displaced cartilage of the knee (locked knee)

This may occur when playing games and a cartilage in the knee is displaced or torn, as from a violent kick that fails to connect, or by slipping on a step, or by twisting the body violently whilst standing on one leg.

Signs and symptoms

These are similar to those of a dislocation, but there is no deformity present, and severe pain is commonly referred to the inner side of the knee;

– the knee is held in a bent position and though further flexion may be possible, it cannot be straightened;

– attempts to straighten the knee causes more severe pain;

– there is usually tenderness over the displaced cartilage;

– fluid to the joint causes swelling.

Treatment

1. Raise and support the leg.
2. Protect the knee with soft padding extending well above and below the joint, and apply a firm bandage, in the most comfortable position for the casualty.
3. Remove to hospital.

CHAPTER TEN

The nervous system and unconsciousness

The nervous system

This consists of two parts –
1. The *Cerebro-spinal system*, and
2. The *Autonomic system*.

These systems control the movements and functions of the body.

Cerebro-spinal system

This consists of the brain, spinal cord and the nerves.

The *brain* is composed of a large number of nerve cells from which nerve fibres, forming a bundle, pass through the base of the skull and enter the spinal column as the *spinal cord*, which continues down to the lower end of the spine. At various points *nerves* leave the spinal cord to reach the different parts of the body to initiate movements of the voluntary muscles and transmit to the brain such sensations as pain, taste, sight, smell, hearing and touch from the various sense organs.

Autonomic system

This consists of a network of nerves which control the involuntary muscles and regulate many vital functions of the body. The autonomic system is not under the control of the will and acts continuously, whether a person is awake or asleep.

Unconsciousness

Unconsciousness is the result of injury to or interference with the functions of the brain. The severity may vary but the following terms are used for certain stages in a progression from consciousness to unconsciousness, or visa versa:

Full consciousness – alert, able to answer questions normally.

Drowsiness – easily roused but relapses into unconsciousness.

Stupor – can be roused only with difficulty: any answers may be unreliable.

Coma – cannot be roused at all.

General rules for treatment

1. Ensure no obstruction to air passages – remove false teeth, clear the mouth of mucus, blood, detached teeth, etc. Provide plenty of fresh air – open windows and doors, keep back crowds. Loosen clothing about neck, chest and waist.
2. If breathing begins to fail or stops, immediately commence artificial respiration.
3. Search for and control any serious bleeding.
4. Establish level of consciousness: record any changes for information of the doctor.

Figure 100: The recovery position.

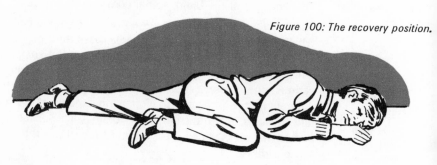

5. Place the casualty in the recovery position (Fig. 100), with head slightly lower than the feet.
6. Cover with a blanket and place one under him if possible.
7. Make arrangements for transport to hospital.
8. If removal to hospital is delayed, check the casualty's responses and pulse rate at intervals, and keep a written record for the doctor.
9. If consciousness returns, speak encouragingly and reassure the casualty: moisten his lips with water.

Do not give drink to an unconscious casualty.

Do not leave him unattended.

Note: Advise any person who has been unconscious for even a moment to see his own doctor.

Treatment cards When examining an unconscious person, carefully search pockets, handbag, etc., if possible in the presence of a reliable witness, for any Treatment Card which may be helpful in deciding on the correct treatment.

Diabetic Card labels the casualty as a diabetic. Sudden dizziness, faintness or coma may be due to excess of insulin.

Steroid Card indicates that the casualty is having some form of cortisone treatment.

Anti-Coagulant Card indicates that the casualty is taking drugs to reduce the clotting of blood.

Medic-Alert Bracelet may be worn, which gives certain medical particulars of the wearer.

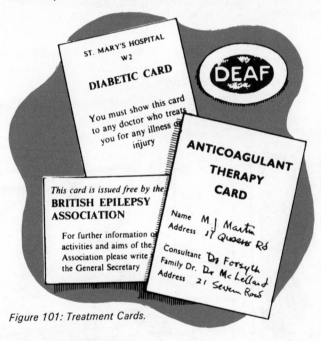

ST. MARY'S HOSPITAL
W 2
DIABETIC CARD
You must show this card
to any doctor who treat
you for any illness o
injury

DEAF

This card is issued free by the
BRITISH EPILEPSY
ASSOCIATION
For further information o
activities and aims of the
Association please write
the General Secretary

ANTICOAGULANT
THERAPY
CARD
Name M. J. Martin
Address 17 Queens Rd
Consultant Dr Forsyth
Family Dr. Dr McLelland
Address 21 Severn Road

Figure 101: Treatment Cards.

Head injury

Injuries to the head may cause wounds of the scalp and fractures of the skull bones, with or without damage to the brain. If there has been damage or disturbance to the brain, consciousness may be clouded or lost. Associated injuries

103

to the spine, chest, abdomen or limbs may be present but masked.

Fracture of the skull

See 'Injuries to Bones', page 82.

Injury to the brain

Damage to the brain may result in cerebral concussion or compression.

Concussion

Is a condition of widespread but temporary disturbance of the brain. 'Brain shaking' is a good description. It may be caused by a blow on the head, a fall from a height onto the feet, or a blow on the point of the jaw.

Signs and symptoms

There is a brief loss of consciousness, with shallow breathing;
— the face is pale with skin cold and clammy;
— the pulse is rapid and weak;
— recovery may be accompanied by nausea and vomiting;
— loss of memory for events just before and after the injury is common.

Note: Should unconsciousness persist, suspect compression.

Compression

There is actual pressure on the brain either by blood or a

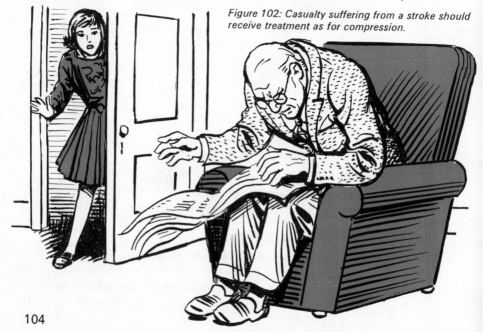

Figure 102: Casualty suffering from a stroke should receive treatment as for compression.

depressed fracture of the skull. The condition may directly follow concussion.

Signs and
Symptoms

In this condition the breathing becomes noisy;
– the face may be flushed with body temperature raised;
– the pulse becomes slow;
– the pupils of the eyes may be unequal in size or dilated, and not react to light;
– there may be weakness or paralysis on one side of the body.

As compression develops, the casualty's level of consciousness falls: this signifies *the most urgent need of medical care.*

Stroke

A similar condition of compression can occur from bleeding into the brain in persons with high blood pressure, often elderly, producing what is known as a 'stroke'. It is accompanied by the same signs as those of compression (Fig. 102), but the absence of signs of injury and a history of high blood pressure help with the diagnosis. The treatment is as for compression.

Concussion or compression

Treatment

Carry out the General Rules for the Treatment of Unconsciousness as far as required.

In the case of concussion, keep careful watch for signs of compression developing.

Epileptic fit

There are two types of epilepsy.

Minor epilepsy

This is of very short duration, when an individual suddenly goes pale, his eyes become fixed or staring, where the unconsciousness is momentary and he recovers quickly with no recollection of what has happened.

Major epilepsy

This is a true epileptic fit –
– the casualty suddenly loses consciousness and falls to the ground;
– becomes rigid for a few seconds with flushed or livid face and neck;

105

– then commences convulsions, alternative contraction an[d] relaxation of groups of muscles;

– noisy breathing with frothing at the mouth, which ma[y] be blood-stained if the tongue has been bitten.

During convulsions, which are frequently quite violent an[d] last for a few minutes, he may lose control of bladder [o]r bowel (incontinence). He then has a pause when he i[s] quite relaxed (flaccid) but is dazed, feels exhausted an[d] often falls into a deep sleep.

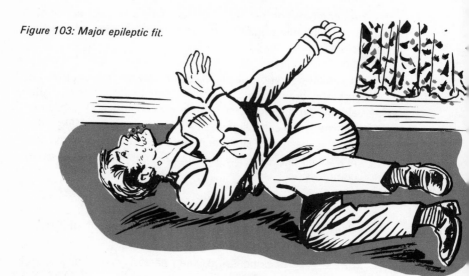

Figure 103: Major epileptic fit.

Treatment

1. Guide the convulsive movements of the casualty in orde[r] to prevent him damaging himself. *Do not* forcibly restrain[ ]but remove any source of danger present.

2. If opportunity occurs, remove any false teeth and put a[ ]knotted handkerchief between his jaws, as far back as[ ]possible, to prevent the tongue being bitten.

3. Keep a careful watch until the convulsions cease and the[ ]casualty recovers consciousness.

4. Advise him to see his doctor, or, if necessary, send him to hospital.

Hysterical fits

These usually occur under emotional stress and may closely simulate an epileptic fit but are more dramatic and staged to appeal to a sympathetic audience. The fits vary from temporary loss of control with shouting and screaming to something more dramatic with arms flung about, crying, tearing at the hair and clothes.

If the First Aider is certain there is no other cause for the condition, he should speak gently but firmly to the casualty and refrain from showing sympathy. He should be referred to medical aid when sufficiently recovered.

Infantile convulsions

These sometimes occur as the result of a raised temperature from any cause, such as the onset of an infectious disease, teething, stomach or chest trouble, throat or ear infection.

There is congestion of the face and neck and froth may appear at the mouth;
– there may be twitching of the muscles;
– stiffness or rigidity with the head and spine arched backwards;
– holding of the breath and eyes turned upwards.

1. Ensure a good supply of fresh air.
2. Loosen tight clothing about the neck, chest and waist.
3. Place the child in the recovery position, if possible: if not with head low and turned to one side.
4. If the child has a high temperature it may be reduced by tepid sponging.
5. Obtain medical aid: reassure the child's parents.

Diabetic emergencies

Two different and opposite conditions may arise –
– Insulin coma – due to excess of insulin.
– Diabetic coma – due to an inadequate supply of insulin.

A diabetic person usually carries a card indicating the treatment he is receiving and also has on him lumps of sugar if on insulin treatment.

There is pallor of the skin with profuse sweating;
– the pulse is rapid and the breathing shallow with no odour to the breath;
– the limbs may tremble;

107

– the casualty may be confused and is sometimes abnormally aggressive. The condition may easily be mistaken for someone who has taken too much alcohol.

– there may be faintness or unconsciousness.

Diabetic coma

The face is flushed and the skin dry;

– the breathing is deep and sighing with the breath smelling strongly of musty apples or nail varnish;

– the casualty passes gradually into a diabetic coma.

It may not be easy to decide whether the casualty is suffering from excess or lack of insulin.

Treatment

If conscious –

Do not hesitate – give drink sweetened with two full tablespoonfuls of sugar, or give lumps of sugar or other sweet substances. If he improves dramatically, the problem is excess of insulin: see that he gets more sugar. If he does not improve, the giving of sugar will cause no harm.

If unconscious –

– place in the recovery position and ***arrange urgent removal to hospital.***

CHAPTER ELEVEN

Burns and scalds

The effect of burns and scalds are similar and their serious-ness depends on many factors, the most important being the part involved and extent rather than the depth of the injury. In young children, especially infants, even small burns should be regarded as serious and hospital treatment sought without delay.

Burns

A burn is caused by –
– **Dry heat** – fire or hot objects, exposure to sun (Fig. 104).
– **Contact with an electric current** or by lightning
– **Friction** from a revolving wheel or fast moving rope
– **Strong acids** and alkalis such as sulphuric acid or caustic soda.

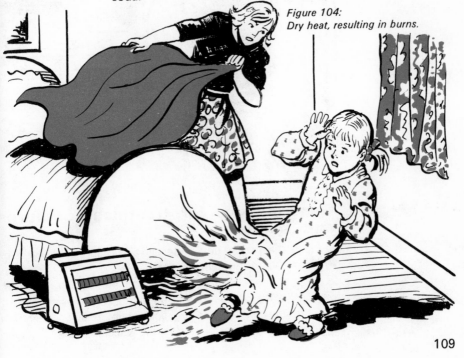

Figure 104:
Dry heat, resulting in burns.

Scalds

A scald is caused by –
Moist heat – such as boiling water or steam.

– Severe pain.
– Reddening of the skin and sometimes blistering. There may be destruction of the skin and deeper tissues.
– Shock, which may be a great danger and increases rapidly with the loss of fluid (plasma) oozing from the burnt surface and from the escape of blood or plasma into the tissues, causing swelling of the part.

Figure 105: Moist heat, resulting in scalds.

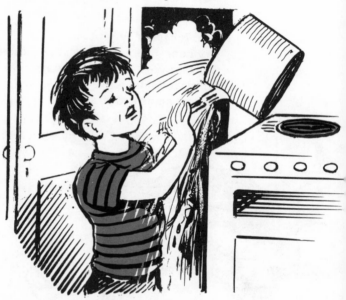

General rules for treatment of burns and scalds

1. Place the part gently under slow running cold water or immerse the part in cool water.
2. Remove promptly anything of a constrictive nature – rings, bangles, belts, boots – before the part starts to swell.
3. Carefully remove clothing soaked in boiling water, but *do not* remove burnt clothing as it will have been rendered

110

sterile by the heat.

4. Cover the injured part with a dressing or freshly laundered linen. With a burn of the face it may be necessary to cut a mask with a hole for breathing.

5. Immobilise a badly burned limb.

6. Give small cold drinks at frequent intervals to a badly injured conscious casualty.

7. *Arrange for immediate removal to hospital of all seriously burned or scalded casualties.*

Do not break blisters.

Clothing on fire

When a person's clothing catches fire, quell the flames and cool the tissues with water or other non-flammable fluid if immediately to hand.

If no such fluid is available, hold a rug in front of yourself for protection and wrap it round the casualty, lay him flat and smother the flames. Nylon and other such material should not be used.

If a person's clothing catches fire when he is alone, he should roll himself in the nearest available wrap to smother the flames, and call for assistance.

Burns and scalds of mouth and throat

These may cause swelling within the throat and this may interfere with breathing.

Treatment

1. *Urgent removal to hospital should be arranged.*
2. The casualty should be placed in the recovery position;
3. If conscious, given sips of cold water to drink.
4. If breathing is failing, give artificial respiration.

Burns caused by corrosive chemicals

1. Flood the part thoroughly and continuously with running water. Make sure the water drains away freely and safely.
2. Remove contaminated clothing as quickly as possible, taking care not to burn yourself.
3. Apply the general rules for the treatment of burns.

Eye injury

An eye may be injured by splashes of a liquid chemical or by solid matter such as lime.

111

Treatment

1. Hold the casualty's head under a gently running tap, or plunge it in a basin of water and instruct him to blink his eye repeatedly.

Figure 106: Washing the eye.

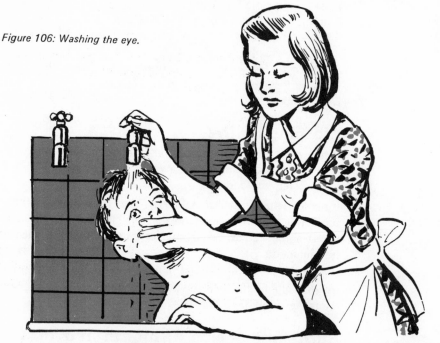

2. Sit or lay the casualty down with head tilted right back and turned towards the affected side. Flush the part copiously with tepid or cool water, gently opening the eyelids with your fingers, protecting the uninjured eye.
If lime has entered the eye, rinse the upper lid and ensure that none is adhering to its surface.
3. Apply a dressing lightly over the eye.
4. ***Arrange urgent removal to hospital.***

Sunburn

This can produce redness of the skin, with swelling and even blistering, giving serious discomfort. People should be warned against over-exposure to the sun, especially when the body is wet with sea water or sweat.

The general rules for the treatment of burns and scalds should be applied when such burns have occured.

112

CHAPTER TWELVE

Poisoning

A poison is any substance, solid, liquid or gas, which when taken into the body in sufficient quantity, is capable of impairing or destroying life.
It may be taken –
– through the lungs
– by the mouth
– by injection under the skin, *or*
– by absorption through the skin.

Through the lungs

This occurs by breathing household gas (not North Sea gas), or fumes from fires, stoves, motor exhausts or smoke. Poisoning from industrial gases may also occur: carbon tetrachloride (in some fire extinguishers and dry cleaning solvents), trichorethylene (in degreasing and dry cleaning agents, and as an anaesthetic.) Hydrogen sulphide, cyanogen gas and cyanide fumes, both of which are rapidly fatal.

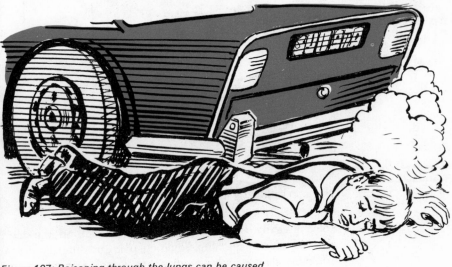

Figure 107: Poisoning through the lungs can be caused by car exhaust gases.

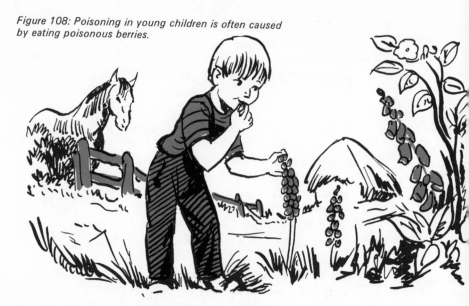

Figure 108: Poisoning in young children is often caused by eating poisonous berries.

Figure 109: Accidental poisoning—taken by mouth.

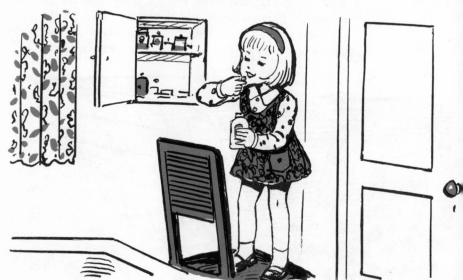

By the mouth   Some swallowed poisons when irritant act on the food passage, causing retching, vomiting, pain and often diarrhoea. Common causes are – poisonous fungi and berries or decomposed food.

Strong acids and alkalis (corrosives) will burn the lips, mouth, gullet and stomach, causing intense pain.

Barbiturates and aspirin (non-corrosives) produced depression, drowsiness and finally coma. Aspirin may also cause vomiting.

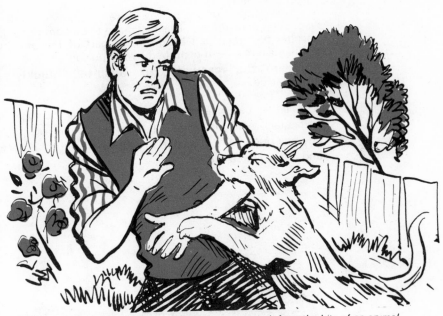

Figure 110: Virus infection can result from the bite of an animal.

By absorption through the skin *Common causes* are certain pesticides used by farmers, such as Parathion, Lindane, etc. They cause convulsions if swallowed.

General rules for the treatment of poisoning

The aim of First Aid is to sustain life and remove the casualty urgently to hospital.

1. If the casualty is conscious—
— ask him quickly what happened; remember he may lose consciousness at any time.

115

If lips and mouth show signs of burns give quantities of water, milk or barley water to dilute the poison.

Remove the casualty to hospital quickly by car or ambulance.

2. If casualty is unconscious

— *if breathing freely*, place him in the recovery position, thus ensuring an open airway;

— *if breathing is failing or has ceased*, commence artificial respiration immediately. This may have to be continued until hospital treatment can be given, as part of the breathing mechanism has been disturbed by the poison.

Remove the casualty to hospital quickly by ambulance.

3. In either case, send to hospital with the casualty, any particulars available, together with any remaining poison, any box or container which may help to identify the poison, and any vomited matter.

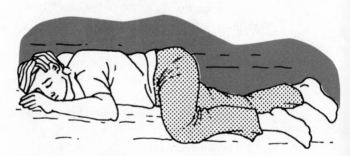

Figure 111: The recovery position

CHAPTER THIRTEEN

Miscellaneous conditions

Extremes of temperature

Excessive cold and heat can cause damage to the skin or body in such a way that tissues locally, or body functions generally, may be so seriously affected that death results.

Locally, cold may cause frostbite at the extremities (fingers, toes, ears and nose), while heat can cause blistering and ulceration of exposed parts.

Effects of cold

The onset is insiduous and may pass unnoticed in those on expeditions or mountaineering. The severity varies with age and the physical condition which governs the ability of the individual to resist. The healthy adult can regulate his body temperature naturally, *except* when over-fatigued by the combination of excercise and anxiety. The term 'exposure' is often used to describe this condition.

Signs and symptoms

There is increasing slowness of physical and mental response;
– stumbling, cramps and shivering;
– difficulties in speech and vision;
– unreasonable behaviour or irritability.

Warning to travellers
If any of these symptoms occur, **take shelter, or improvise it, and rest.**
It is essential –
– to prevent further loss of body heat;
– to overcome exhaustion;
– to obtain help if possible.

Treatment

At the site –
1. Protect the casualty from wind or sleet.
2. If possible, wrap him in dry clothing; put him in a sleeping bag.
3. Give warm sweet drinks, e.g. condensed milk.

At the base –

Rapid rewarming in a hot bath, bringing the temperature up to 42-45°C (107-113°F).

Note: **All cases** of prolonged exposure to cold should be considered as serious and in urgent need of medical care.

Severe accidental cooling of the body (hypothermia)

This is a dangerous lowering of the body temperature which may occur at any age, but especially in babies and the elderly who lack the ability to regulate their own temperature, even when not fatigued.

Causes

Exposure to cold:
– from weather or in an unheated house;
– prolonged immersion in water;
– lowering of the sensibility of cold by alcohol, drugs and poisoning.

A contributory cause may be a medical condition such as diabetes or diarrhoea.

Infants. Babies must be kept constantly warm during the first few weeks as they cannot yet regulate their own body temperature.

Elderly and infirm. Those living alone, especially pensioners on an inadequate diet, may be found collapsed in a state of stupor on the floor, or lying in bed. In each case they may be fully clothed and the condition could be mistaken for a 'stroke' or heart attack.

Signs and Symptoms

Infants are quiet and refuse food. The healthy appearance of pink face, hands and feet is deceptive, because they are quite cold to the touch.

Elderly and infirm are pale and in a state of collapse;
– the casualty is deadly cold to the touch;
– the pulse is slow, weak or imperceptible;
– the breathing is slow and shallow.

Treatment

1. Place the casualty between blankets and allow to warm up **gradually**.
2. If conscious, give tepid or warm sweet drinks.

Do not use hot water bottles or electric blankets as these will cause sudden dilatation of the superficial blood vessels taking away blood from the essential organs, thus causing a fatal drop in the casualty's blood pressure and temperature.

Frostbite

This occurs most commonly if a part of the body is exposed to the wind in very cold weather. The ears, nose, chin, fingers and toes are most frequently affected.

Signs and symptoms

Feeling and power of movement may be lost;
– to the casualty the affected part may feel cold, painful and stiff;
– there is blanching and numbness of the part which, if not properly and promptly treated, may lead to gangrene.

Treatment

1. Take care of the casualty's general condition by sheltering him from the weather, and give warm drinks.
2. Remove promptly anything of a constrictive nature – gloves, rings, boots.
3. Thaw the affected part without the use of heat – *do not* use hot water bottles, fires or friction –
If the area is the **face,** cover with a dry gloved hand until colour and sensation are restored;
– if a **hand,** place under the clothing in his armpits;
– if the **feet,** wrap them in a warm blanket or sleeping bag.
4. *Transport the casualty to medical aid as quickly as possible.*

Effects of excessive heat

Heat exhaustion

The most vulnerable are those unacclimatised to high temperature and humidity.

Signs and symptoms

The onset is gradual and it is caused by exposure to excessive heat, especially moist heat. Fluid and salt loss is considerable from excessive sweating and is often aggravated by a gastrointestinal upset with diarrhoea and vomiting.

Muscular cramps from salt deficiency is an early sign.
– the casualty is exhausted and may be restless;
– his face is pale and cold with a clammy sweat;
– the pulse and breathing are rapid;
– he may complain of headache, dizziness and nausea;
– any sudden movement may cause him to faint.

Treatment	1. Lay the casualty down in a cool place.
	2. If conscious give cold water to drink to which has been added a half-a-teaspoonful of common salt to each pint (half a litre) of water.
	3. If unconscious, place in the recovery position.

Heat stroke

Onset is more sudden and this condition may be preceded by heat exhaustion.

It may be brought on by a high atmospheric temperature with a hot drying wind or by high humidity and lack of air current.

It may also be caused by an acute debilitating illness, such as malaria.

Signs and symptoms

Unconsciousness comes on quickly;
– the face is flushed, the skin hot and dry;
– the pulse full and bounding;
– the breathing noisy;
– the casualty may be confused, stuporous or in a coma;
– a temperature of 40°C (104°F) or more may occur.

Treatment

1. Quickly strip the casualty and wrap in a cold wet sheet, keeping it wet until the casualty's temperature has been lowered to 38°C (101°F).
2. Place him in the recovery position.
3. Direct currents of air on the casualty from above and below by hand or by electric fans.
4. On recovery, cover the casualty with a dry sheet and, if possible, get him into air-conditioned accommodation.
5. Send to hospital.

Note: If the casualty's temperature rises again, repeat the treatment.

Cramp

This consists of involuntary shortening of a muscle or group of muscles, which may be caused by poor co-ordination during exercise, by chilling as in swimming or by excessive loss of salt and body fluids from severe sweating, diarrhoea, etc.

Treatment

The shortened muscle must be stretched.

In the hand – forcibly, but gently, straighten out the fingers.

120

In the thigh – straighten the knee and raise the leg with one hand under the heel while pressing down the knee with the other hand.

In the calf or foot – straighten the knee and with the hand forcibly draw the foot up towards the shin; *or*

– straighten the toes and get the casualty to stand on the ball of the foot.

Salt deficiency – give copious drafts of cold water to which has been added half a-teaspoonful of common salt to a pint (half a litre) of water.

Foreign body in the eye

Particles of grit, loose lashes, insects and small fragments of metal or glass, etc., may lodge in the eyeball, or under the eyelid causing considerable discomfort and inflammation, if not speedily removed.

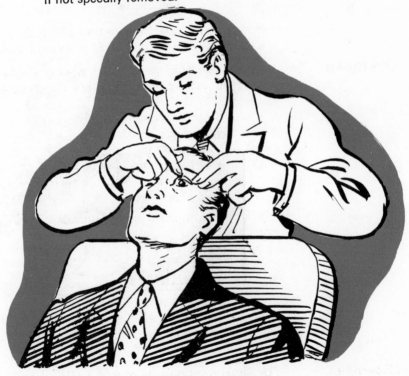

Figure 112: Removal of foreign body from the eye.

Treatment

1. Prevent the casualty from rubbing his eye.

2. *Do not* attempt to remove the foreign body if it is
– on the pupil of the eye, *or*
– embedded or adherent to the eyeball.

Cover the eye with a soft pad of cotton wool, secure lightly in position, and seek medical aid, *otherwise*

3. Seat him facing the light. Instruct him to look up and pull down the lower lid and, if the foreign body is visible, remove it with the corner of a clean handkerchief or material which has been soaked in a little water.

4. If the foreign body is under the upper lid, ask the casualty to look down, grasp the eyelashes and pull the upper lid downwards and outwards over the lower lid. This may dislodge the foreign body. If not, ask the casualty to blink his eye under water.

5. If the foreign body is of a poisonous or corrosive nature, prolonged irrigation of the eye is necessary; see page 112.

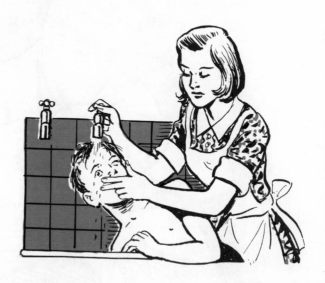

If still unsuccessful and medical aid is not immediately available –

(i) stand behind the casualty resting his head against your chest, and ask him to look down;

122

(*ii*) place a smooth matchstick at the base of the upper lid and press it gently backwards;

(*iii*) grasp the lashes and turn the lid over the matchstick, so everting the eyelid (Fig. 112).

(*iv*) remove the foreign body with the corner of a clean handkerchief or material which has been soaked in a little water.

Injuries to the eyeball

Treatment

The eye may be involved in a wound or a crush injury.

1. Lay the casualty down at absolute rest.
2. Place a soft pad of cotton wool over the closed eye, secure lightly in position.
3. **Remove to hospital as soon as possible.**

Strong acid or alkali in the eye

For treatment see 'Injuries from Corrosive Chemicals', page 111.

Foreign body in the ear canal

Insects: Flood the ear with tepid water or olive oil (Fig. 113). The insect will float out.

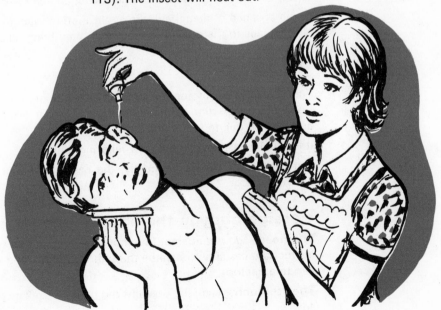

Figure 113: Flooding the ear with olive oil or tepid water.

123

Beads, beans, etc.: *do not* attempt to remove but take the casualty, usually a child, to a doctor or hospital.

Bleeding from the ear

If from a laceration of the **outer ear,** control by direct pressure over a dressing or other clean material.

If from the **ear canal** –
– *after a head injury,* suspect a fracture of the skull;
– *after a blow or blast,* suspect a rupture of the eardrum.

Treatment

See 'Treatment of Bleeding from Special Areas'. page 67

Earache

This may occur suddenly due to a sudden change of pressure on the drum during air travel or in underwater swimming.

Treatment

The casualty should try and equalise the pressure by holding his nose, at the same time swallowing, or blowing out his cheeks.

If the ear is inflamed, obtain medical aid immediately.

Toothache

This is often causes distress and needs dental treatment.

In the absence of dental aid, the application of warmth and oil of cloves to the offending tooth will often bring relief.

Headache

This is always a symptom of some other condition. It occurs frequently when the temperature rises, or from eyestrain and is often due to worry and stress.

It is usually eased by a mild pain-relieving tablet.

If it persists or occurs frequently, the casualty should see his own doctor.

Foreign body in the nose or stomach

The nose – *do not* attempt to remove the foreign body, but instruct the casualty to breathe through his mouth, and take him to a doctor.

The stomach – calm the casualty and parents; seek medical advice.

Do not give anything by the mouth.

Rupture (abdominal hernia)

This is a protrusion of some part of the abdominal contents through the muscular wall of the abdomen under the skin. It occurs most frequently in the groin or through the scar of an abdominal operation.

It causes a painless swelling which comes on after exercise, lifting heavy objects, coughing or straining on the lavatory when constipated.

The condition may come on suddenly with a swelling, pain and possibly vomiting. A 'strangulated hernia', when a piece of the bowel is nipped, may present these signs and symptoms and is an urgent surgical problem.

Treatment
1. Reassure the casualty.
2. Lay him down and support the head and shoulders, bend and support his knees.
3. If vomiting occurs or seems likely, place him in the recovery position.
4. Seek medical aid.

Do not attempt to reduce the swelling.

Asthma

Sudden attacks of difficult breathing often occur at night and the casualty has difficulty in forcing air out of his lungs.

Treatment
1. Place him in a comfortable position, usually sitting up or leaning forward resting on a table or pillow, keeping his back straight.
2. Reassure him and provide plenty of fresh air.
3. Obtain medical aid or send to hospital.

Hiccups

Commonly the result of digestive disturbance or 'nervousness'.

Relief is frequently obtained by sips of cold water, or by holding the breath.

If the condition persists for more than a few hours, the casualty's doctor should be informed.

Stings and bites

Stings

These can be either from animals, insects or plants.

In insect stings –

Treatment

1. Remove the sting, if present, using forceps or tweezers, or a point of a needle which has been sterilised by passing it through a flame and allowing it to cool.

2. Apply surgical spirit, a weak solution of ammonia or bicarbonate of soda.

3. If the sting is in the mouth, give a mouthwash of bicarbonate of soda – one teaspoonful to a tumbler of water. If there is difficulty in breathing, place the casualty in the recovery position and give ice to suck. Seek medical aid immediately.

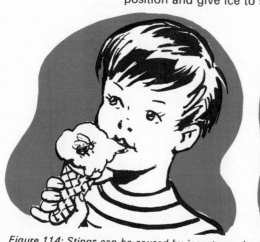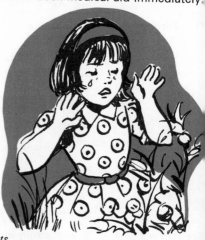

Figure 114: Stings can be caused by insects or plants.

Bites

In countries where rabies may be present, all dog bite cases should be referred to medical aid.

Animal bites are treated as ordinary wounds.

Snake bites

Snakes will not usually attack unless stepped on or cornered. Some snakes are poisonous and their bite is dangerous and may be fatal.

Snake bites are greatly feared and this fear increases the degree of shock to the casualty.

In those countries where dangerous snakes are common, anti-snake serum is kept available in known centres. If the snake is killed, it should be kept for identification.

126

1. Calm and reassure the casualty; lay him down, keep at complete rest.
2. Flush the wound with soapy water and wash away all venom that has oozed from the wound.
3. Support and immobilise the limb.
4. Obtain medical aid as soon as possible.
5. Should breathing begin to fail, commence artificial respiration.

'Winding'

Due to a blow in the upper part of the abdomen (*Solar plexus*) which may cause fainting or even collapse.

1. Place the casualty in the recovery position.
2. Loosen tight clothing at the neck, chest and waist.
3. Gently massage the upper abdomen.

Stitch

A painful spasm of the diaphragm, often occurring on exertion when not in training.

It is relieved by rest, sips of hot water, and gently rubbing of the affected side.

CHAPTER FOURTEEN

Handling and transport of injured persons

It is important in the early stages of any accident to decide whether the casualty should be treated where the accident occurred or whether, by moving him, it would be safer and easier to carry out a complete examination and treatment. If the casualty is seriously injured or if he has multiple injuries, it may be better to deal with him where he lies, as much further damage can be caused in removal. A First Aider acting alone or with unskilled help, may easily cause more damage trying to move the casualty than by dealing with him at the site of the accident.

Examination Before moving a casualty, unless life is endangered by fire, falling debris or a poisoned atmosphere, it is important, especially if he is unconscious, to carry out a quick but systematic examination of the head and neck, chest and abdomen and all limbs, which, if injured, must be supported during removal.

After the initial removal from danger, or to enable treatment to be carried out more satisfactorily, *do not* forget to carry out the remainder of the examination. Two of the commonest mistakes made in first aid practice are –
– to move the casualty without making a proper preliminary examination so that insufficient or incorrect support is given during removal; or
– after removal, to forget to complete the examination of the casualty because a preliminary examination was made.

In either case, additional damage may be caused to the casualty because certain injuries may have been missed.

Removal An injured or sick person may be removed to shelter by –
1. Support of a single helper.
2. Handseats and the 'kitchen-chair' carry.
3. Blanket lift.

4. Stretcher.

5. Wheeled transport (ambulance).

6. Air and sea travel.

The method to be adopted, and it may be necessary to use more than one, will depend upon –

– the nature and severity of the injury;

– the number of helpers and facilities available;

– the distance to shelter;

– the nature of the route to be covered.

Treatment

The aim of First Aid treatment is to enable a casualty to reach his destination without his condition becoming worse. Therefore –

1. the position assumed by the casualty or in which he has been placed, if generally satisfactory, must not be altered unnecessarily;

2. throughout transport a careful watch must be kept on –

– the general condition of the casualty;

– the maintenance of an open airway;

– the control of bleeding and the continuous immobilisation of fractures and large wounds;

3. transport must be safe and steady.

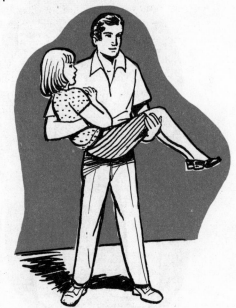

Figure 115: A cradle.

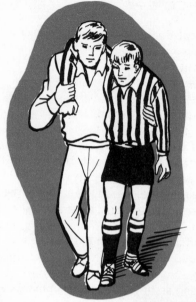

Figure 116: Human crutch.

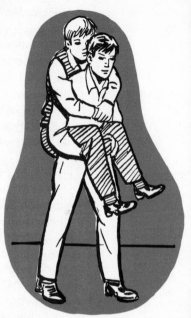

Figure 117: Pick-a-back.

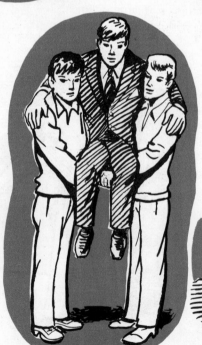

Figure 118: The four-handed seat with detail of hand grip.

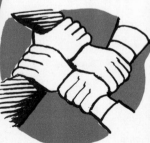

One First Aider only
1. *Cradle* (Fig. 115)
2. *Human crutch* (Fig. 116)
3. *Pick-a-back* (Fig. 117).

Two or more First Aiders
1. *The four-handed seat* (Fig. 118).
Two First Aiders grasp their own left wrists with their right hand and each others' right wrists with their left hand. Both step off with outside feet and walk forward with ordinary paces.

2. *The two-handed seat* (Fig. 119 and 120)
Two First Aiders, one on each side of the casualty, pass their forearms nearest the casualty under his back just below the shoulders, and pass their other forearms under the middle of his thighs, when they clasp hands using the hook-grip (Fig. 121). To prevent hurting by the finger nails, a folded handkerchief should be placed between the palms of the

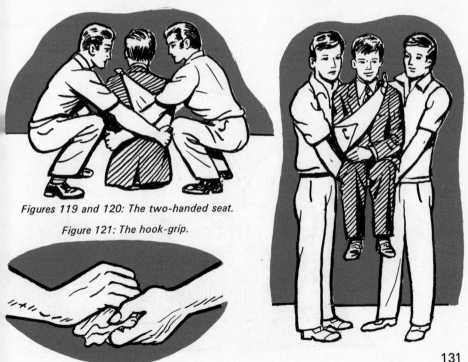

Figures 119 and 120: The two-handed seat.

Figure 121: The hook-grip.

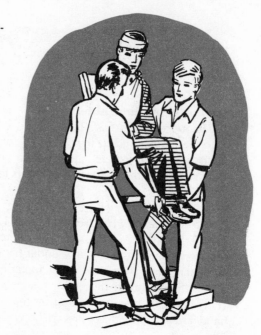

Figure 122: The kitchen-chair method.

bearers. Both step off with outside feet and walk forward with ordinary paces.

3. *The 'kitchen-chair' carry* (Fig. 122)

Blanket lift

The placing of a casualty onto a blanket is described on page 85 (Fig. 123).

Figure 123: Blanket lift – positioning the blanket.

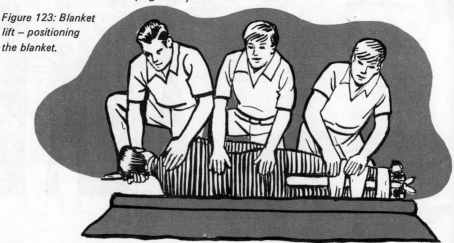

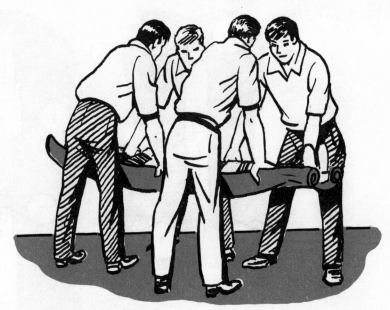

Figure 124: Blanket lift.

When lifting by a blanket, the edges are rolled up close to the casualty's sides and lifted as shown in Fig. 124.

Stretchers

Stretchers in common use are of two patterns – 'ordinary' (Fig. 125) and 'telescopic handled'.

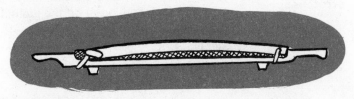

Figure 125: Ordinary stretcher.

In principle they are alike, the difference being that the handles of the second type can be pushed under the poles. thus reducing the overall length to six feet.

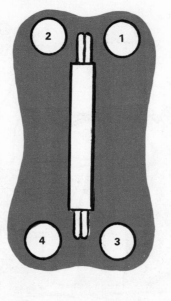

Figures 126 and 127:
Positioning of bearers.

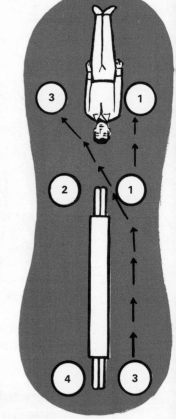

Positioning of Bearers
See Figs. 126 and 127.

Preparing and blanketing a stretcher

The stretcher is opened out and the traverse bars fully opened. The stretcher should be tested by one person lying on it and each end raised off the ground in turn.

Blanketing with one blanket
See Fig. 128.

Blanketing with two blankets
See Fig. 129.

Loading a stretcher

1. *When the casualty is not lying on a blanket and none is available,* bearers will take up positions (Fig. 130). Using the hook-grip (Fig. 121), No. 1 joins his left hand with the left hand of No. 4 and his right hand with the right hand of No. 3. No. 4 supports the head and shoulders, No. 2 the lower limbs (Fig. 131). The casualty is carefully and evenly

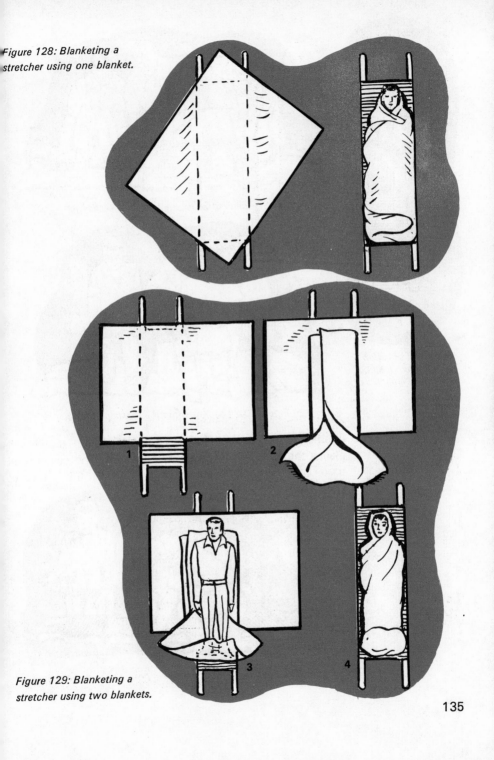

Figure 128: Blanketing a stretcher using one blanket.

Figure 129: Blanketing a stretcher using two blankets.

135

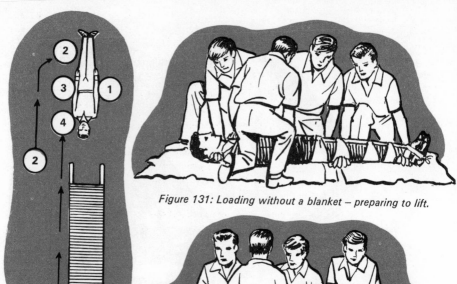

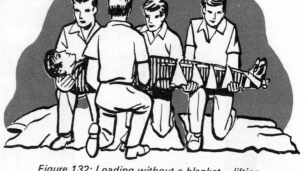

Figure 131: Loading without a blanket — preparing to lift.

Figure 132: Loading without a blanket — lifting.

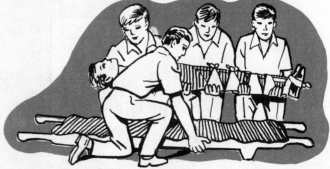

Figure 130: Position of bearers when loading without a blanket.

lifted on to the knees of Nos. 2, 3 and 4 (Fig. 132), then No. 1 places the stretcher in position (Fig. 133). The casualty is then carefully and evenly lowered on to the stretcher (Fig. 134).

Figure 133: Loading without blanket — positioning of the stretcher.

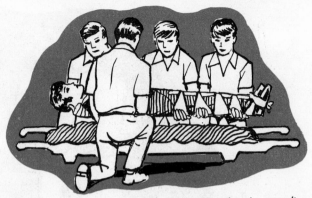

Figure 134: Loading without blanket – lowering the casualty.

2. *When the casualty is lying on a blanket*, bearers will place themselves on each side of the casualty, Nos. 1 and 2 at the feet, Nos. 3 and 4 at the head. The edges of the blanket are rolled against the side of the casualty and each bearer firmly grasps the rolled edges. At the command of No. 1, the casualty is carefully and evenly raised and, unless there is a fifth person present to push the stretcher under the casualty, the bearers will take short side steps until the casualty is over the stretcher. He is then gently lowered on to it.

Lifting a casualty with three bearers
Two bearers on their knees, lock their hands in the hook-grip

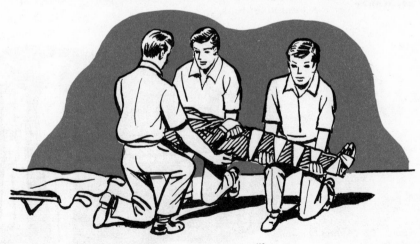

Figure 135: Position for three-bearer lift.

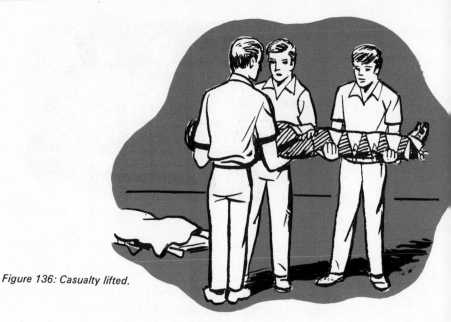

Figure 136: Casualty lifted.

under the casualty's shoulders and hips, the third bearer supports the lower limbs (Fig. 135). They rise together (Fig. 136) and move evenly over the stretcher, lowering the casualty carefully on to it.

Carrying a stretcher

Four-handed carriage (Fig. 137). Each bearer steps off with the inner foot.

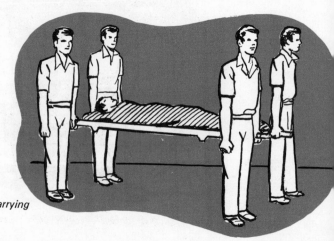

Figure 137: Method of carrying stretcher – four bearers.

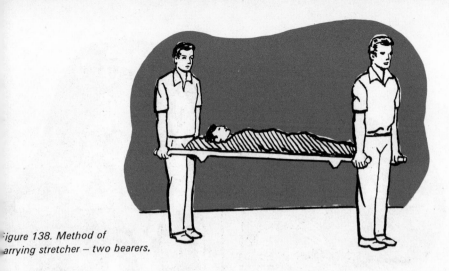

Figure 138. Method of carrying stretcher – two bearers.

Two-handed carriage (Fig. 138). The front bearer steps off with his left foot, the rear bearer with his right.

Improvised stretchers

A stretcher may be improvised in various ways –
– turn the sleeves of two or more coats inside out, pass two poles through them and button up the coats;
– make holes in the bottom corners of two sacks, pass poles through them;
– tie broad bandages at intervals to two poles;
– a hurdle, door or shutter covered with rags, clothing, etc. may also be used and carried as in Fig. 139.

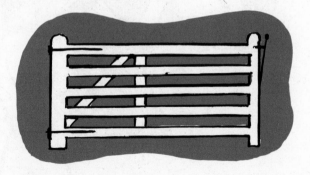

Always test improvised stretchers before use.

139

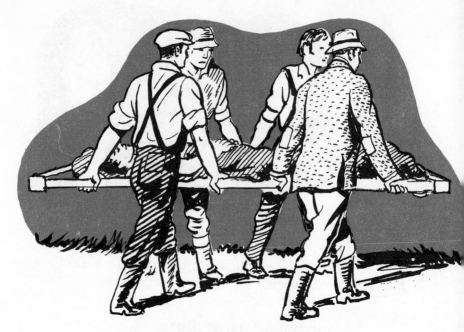

Figure 139: An improvised stretcher.

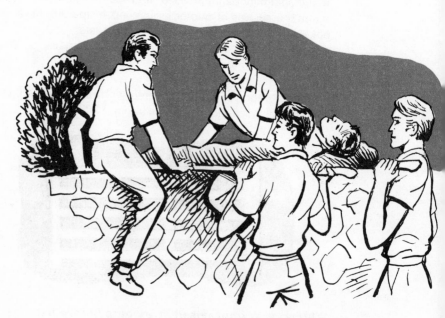

Figure 140: Method of crossing a raised obstruction.

Crossing a wall	Raise the stretcher and lift it on to the wall. Two bearers cross the wall, the stretcher is moved forward and the remaining two bearers cross the wall. The stretcher is then lowered to the ground and the bearers again take up their positions. (Fig. 140).
Crossing a ditch	Using the rear and front handles in succession as weight carriers on the rear and front edges of the ditch, the bearers descend in pairs successively and pass the stretcher forward until the whole is grounded on the far side.

Loading an ambulance

The loaded stretcher is lowered with its head one pace from the doors of the ambulance. With two bearers on each side of the stretcher, it is lifted to the level of the compartment to be loaded, the front bearers ensuring that the stretcher runners are engaged securely in the grooves before relinquishing any part of the weight. The stretcher is then evenly pushed onto its place.

Many ambulances are provided with upper and lower berths. In such cases the sequence of loading is upper right, upper left, lower right, lower left.

Road Accidents

Priorities

If you are clear about the priorities in an accident (that is, th order in which things are done) you are well on the way t being a First Aider. The following are the priorities:

Danger

If you do not deal with threatened danger you and you casualties may be killed. *PILE-UPS* and *FIRE* are th dangers in a road accident: .

Get someone to flag down the traffic far enough away t secure compliance.

Switch off the engine.

Impose a 'No Smoking' ban.

Breathing

A crash victim is often unconscious and cannot breathe because of a kink in his airway.

Open the airway up by extending the head backwards.

Check for obstruction to airway and relieve it.

If still not breathing pinch nose, hold head back and inflate lungs by blowing.

Bleeding

Grasp sides of wound.

Elevate if possible.

Continue pressure on sides of wound with pad and firm bandage.

Coma

You must keep the unconscious patient alive until the ambulance arrives:

Keep the airway open.

Turn into the coma or recovery position.

Watch the airway.

WATCH THE AIRWAY.

Shock

In severe injuries the patient will die in a few hours unless he gets a blood transfusion.

Send for the ambulance with extreme urgency.

Fractures	Immobilise using common sense. Upper limb: use arm sling or pin sleeve to lapel. Lower limb: tie to sound leg after padding between knees and ankles.
Wounds	Stop bleeding. Clean around wound with throw-away tissues. Cover with sterile or clean dressing. Immobilise.
Moving the casualty	Don't, unless you have to (e.g., if the car catches fire or you want to treat one of the priority conditions such as asphyxia or severe bleeding).
Dealing with victims	As soon as you get to the crashed vehicles turn off the ignition and lights to prevent fire. If the victims of the crash are hurt but not bleeding profusely, leave them in the car(s) until trained help comes. *DON'T TWIST, TURN OR MOVE THEM.* If they are lying on the road, cover them with a blanket or coat, leave them there and take steps to guard them from the traffic. Even a victim with a broken back can usually be saved if allowed to lie unmoved. But well meaning people lift them out of the crashed vehicles, bundle them into the back seats of their cars and rush them to hospital – with serious results.
If people are pinned	Often victims otherwise unhurt appear to be trapped when they are merely held by a foot twisted under a seat. If so, crawl in and gently release the foot. *MAKE SURE THE CAR WILL NOT ROLL WHILE YOU DO THIS.*
Sending for the ambulance	Dial 999 and ask for the ambulance service, stating: Where to come. How many patients. The nature of the injuries.

Glossary

Angulation – With regard to fractures. Having an angle or sharp bend where one should not be.

Anti-Coagulant – Drugs used to counteract the clotting of blood. Example: Heparin.

Atrium – L. central court of Roman house. Upper main chambers of the heart (formerly known as left and right Auricles).

Autonomic – Independent: Autonomic nervous system regulates and controls organs and glands which are not under voluntary control.

Bacteria – Modern medical term for germs: the minute living micro-organisms which cause disease in our bodies.

Beatitude – Blessing. See Matthew v. 3-11.

Coma – State of unconsciousness resembling heavy sleep.

Coronary Obstruction – Coronary thrombosis-blockage of the artery supplying the heart.

Cyanosis – Bluish colour seen in face, lips and extremities when the blood in circulation is deficient in oxygen.

Fibrin – A protein formed from the fibrinogen of blood plasma when blood clots.

Floater – When applied to a bandage, indicates that the site varies with the position of the fracture.

Haemoptysis – Bleeding from the lungs, bright red and frothy. May be caused by either injury or disease such as tuberculosis.

Horizontal – Parallel to a flat or level surface, e.g. floor.

Hypothermia – Dangerous lowering of body temperature. Temperatures of 97°F (36°C) and below are considered sub-normal.

Incontinence – Inability to hold urine, faeces, etc., due to loss of muscle control.

Loin – The area of the body bounded by the upper edge of the pelvis and the lower edge of the false ribs on either side of the spinal column.

Maxillo-Facial – As applied to injury implies involvement of the jaw as well as face.

Neil-Robertson Stretcher – Special stretcher of bamboo and canvas designed for use in cramped or confined spaces, especially at sea, holds of ships, etc., in which a jacket type fastening enfolds the body of the casualty and is strapped in place. Rope rings and handles permit easy hoisting and handling.

Oedema – The collection of fluid in the tissues and cavities of the body, as in dropsy.

Pancreas – Digestive gland near stomach secreting insulin.

Paradoxical (breathing) – The opposite to general accepted practice. The chest wall appears to move *inwards* when air is drawn *inwards* into the lungs.

Photophobia – Inability to stand exposure of the eyes to light. Extreme sensitiveness to light.

Plasma – Colourless blood lymph.

Platelets – Cells in the blood concerned with the clotting process.

Porosity – The quality of being porous; full of pores.

Pott's Fracture – Fracture of bone outer side of leg 2 to 3 inches above ankle.

Pupil – The aperture in the centre of the iris of the eye, which admits light to the retina. Varies in size with the intensity of light.

Rabies – Hydrophobia: an acute infectious disease caused by the bite of mad animals (dogs, wolves) transmitted by the saliva.

Semi-Recumbent – Position of casualty in bed or couch reclining with back propped up with two or more pillows, rugs, etc.

Serum – Straw-coloured liquid left when the remainder of blood clots.

Spasm – A convulsive movement or painful contraction of a muscle in any part of the body

144

so that that part cannot continue to work normally.

Spleen – Organ which controls certain blood changes. Once thought to regulate the temperature.

Stertorous – Breathing of a snoring type occurs in cerebral compression and apoplexy, also in state of coma as it does in ordinary sleep, from a relaxed cdndition of the soft palate, which vibrates with the current of air.

Tetanus – Infection affecting the muscles which may contract spasmodically, hence lockjaw.

U.H.V. (Ultra High Voltage) – The high voltage electric supplies for overhead electric traction for British Rail 25,000 volt, 50 cycle AC and 400,000 volt supplies from pylons and overhead cables.

Ventricular – Pertaining to the ventricles: the two lower main chambers of the heart *Auricular* is sometimes used in a similar manner in connection with the two upper main chambers, formerly known as Auricles, but more properly now as the *Atrium*. Hence *Atrial* for matters pertaining to it.

List of illustrations

LIST OF ILLUSTRATIONS

Index

NDEX

INDEX

INDEX

NOTES

NOTES

NOTES